THE SANCTUARY OF ILLNESS

THE SANCTUARY OF ILLNESS

A Memoir of Heart Disease

Carole — With friendship in the memoir form.

Thomas Larson

Thomas Larson
10.31.15.

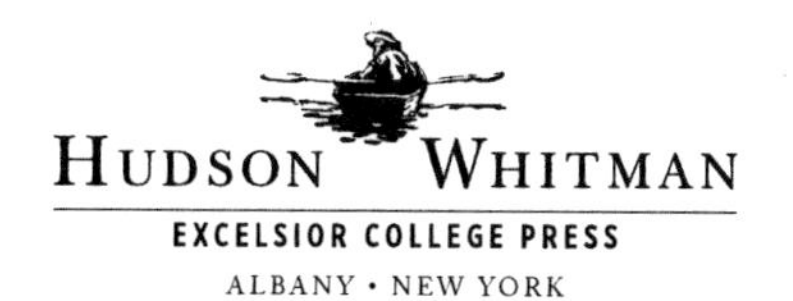

HUDSON WHITMAN
EXCELSIOR COLLEGE PRESS
ALBANY • NEW YORK

The Sanctuary of Illness draws on material from the following previously published essays by Thomas Larson:

"Disenthralled: An End to My Heart Disease"
River Teeth: A Journal of Nonfiction Narrative
Volume 13, Number 2, Spring 2012

"One Way It Happens"
Brevity: A Journal of Concise Literary Nonfiction
January 2013, Issue 41

"Stress Echo"
The Yale Journal for Humanities in Medicine
June 27, 2013

This book is not intended as a substitute for the medical advice of physicians. The reader should regularly consult a physician in matters relating to his/her health and particularly with respect to any symptoms that may require diagnosis or medical attention.

Published by Hudson Whitman/Excelsior College Press
7 Columbia Circle, Albany, NY 12203
www.hudsonwhitman.com

Printed in the United States of America
Book design by Melissa Mykal Batalin
Cover design by Phil Pascuzzo

PCN: 2013948929
ISBN: 978-0-9768813-8-4

To my father, who died of heart disease at sixty-one.

To my older brother, Steve, who died of the same at forty-two.

To my younger brother, Jeff, who, fearing cardiovascular illness, lost seventy-five pounds before his sixtieth birthday.

And to Suzanna—
I wonder, after all our revisions, whether you see yourself in this memoir: weaving you into my story so it becomes *ours* is the hardest felt writing I've ever done, bar none.

As long as humans feel threatened and helpless,
they will seek the sanctuary that illness provides.
—Dr. Robert R. Rynearson

ONE

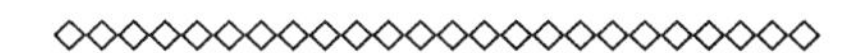

. . . this monster, the body, this miracle, its pain . . .

— Virginia Woolf, "On Being Ill"

Christ, Not Now • It's March, I'm at home in San Diego and getting ready to teach my Monday evening class. It's strange: in the hour prior, I'm hot, sweaty. Constipated. Confused. Breathless, having just lumbered up the stairs to Suzanna's and my bedroom. The second story—how many times have I done that? I tell myself it's work, it's stress, nothing else. I'm out of shape, easily winded. Indeed, for months, I've been trudging on the treadmill, a lot slower than usual. But I'm not sick. I'm older. What age? I have to remember. Fifty-six. Driving to class, I'm heating up, rolling down the window for a breeze. At class, I'm no better. I give my flock a writing assignment, which I check, moving from student to student. Ten minutes pass this way. Then I excuse myself—a quick bathroom stint, I think, should dispel this acidic burn in my throat. I lean into the toilet, try to vomit. Nothing. I crap, blow-it-out like bird shit. That's got it. I rush back to class, wondering what's happening? I don't know. I do know I *don't* want to suffer in the way I'm suffering right now. How will I make it through the next three hours? I've never left in the middle of a class, and only twice in fifteen years have I canceled—the day my mother died and the day one of my twin sons left home, leaving a cryptic note that terrified Suzanna and me. I rationalize it—tonight's lesson needs completing. It's amateurish to postpone the work. Maybe I can do ten minutes on each essay we've read and let them go. From my notes, I outline on the board the writing strategies in each piece. And here it gets strange. The taste of reflux soils my mouth. I feel as though I've just plunged off a cliff and halted midair. Afloat, I sense there is no future: however many years are telescoped into these few minutes. *Years into minutes.* A spiral appears, widens, pinwheels, and sucks me in. I recall how I've told students it's a copout to say, "It felt like an eternity" or "Time dragged on" or "Hours rushed by." Clichés, I've called them. How *do* you capture trauma, intensity, in words? There's no other side to this thought. I discuss one essay in two minutes, the next in a minute, the next, in thirty seconds. My words are boggy, slow. Then I hear myself speak—as though I've been called on—"I'm afraid I'm not feeling well. I have to leave." In my bag, I stuff books and papers. My hands sweat. My legs quake. "For next week," I say—and stop. Everyone is looking at me. "I have to leave." I'm running.

Clothes Off • A nurse takes me to an emergency room bay. "Symptoms?" she asks. "I think I'm having a heart attack," I say again. She tells me to get undressed. I'm sitting on the bed, and begin taking my clothes off—*peeling*, that's the word. They've been stuck on me like a soiled diaper for half an hour. My body is leaking its insides. It's not the soul coming out, wet and furious. It's my skin, like packaging, trying to strip itself of the invader. These goddamn clothes nag because they curtain my fat, a lifelong source of shame. For several years I've gained weight (again)—in the 1980s, a runner, I was svelte; in the 1990s, I got so sedentary and lazy teaching full-time I put the pounds back on; now, in the 2000s, a full-time writer/journalist, and I procrastinate getting back in shape, my belly jellying, a midlife bulge pushing me to 220. I hate the weight. I hate unbuttoning the faded pink travel shirt I've worn for years. I hate unclasping the stretchy waistband pants, size 40, all this so pungent, so whiny—I don't want to see the tumescence over my too-tight underwear: how often I hide behind a T-shirt prior to sex with Suzanna (What sex? It's been months). Why don't I stop worrying? "Stay here," the nurse says, "I'm coming right back." As if I'm going anywhere.

Where is the drug to curb/redirect this avalanche?

Where are my saviors?

I put on the gown. To hell with the ties. I get back on the long plastic mat.

An orderly enters, wires me up to the ECG machine, prints out a graph-paper page on which I espy its Himalayan-like peaks and valleys. He hustles out. He returns. With a well-groomed pro, the Doc, in crisply tailored whites, who tells me what I've known now for an hour: "You're right, Mr. Larson. You're having a heart attack."

I'm Sorry • Is it then that the nurse asks the mandatory questions—my name, my address, my date of birth, my cardiac history (do I say, father, brother, both dead: *of heart attacks*, or the less volatile, *heart disease*), my symptoms (I'm dizzy, I'm hot, my chest aches): Have you ever had angina before, a sudden name for the pain that keeps washing through me? Does she lean over next and smirk a tad wickedly and say, "Please try and relax," and I laugh? Does it happen a minute later that she rifles a medical bag for aspirin and a sublingual nitroglycerin tablet, and asks, almost like an afterthought, who to phone, and I say, *Suzanna*? While I wait, harried and calmed by the theatrical flurry, the pinging machines, the seismic readouts, you appear, curtain-parting and padding your way up to the bed where I lie and where on your face I see two women, you who are unafraid to approach me, indeed, desire my trouble, and you who are shocked to come any closer—

To both of you I say, "I'm sorry."

"Don't be," you reply.

"But I am."

"What for?"

Good question.

I'm sorry that this dread wants *you*, as well as me, to bear it.

Don't Drive Yourself • But I did. My last act of volition. Isn't that why I'm alive and being helped? I got here lickety-split. For which I think I should receive some credit. Ah, we're dialoguing. I'm out of danger. Indeed, I'm purring and holding onto Suzanna, who smiles at the busy, fraught nurse—Suzanna, a psychotherapist, whom I've been with for seventeen years (our home offices adjoin), who is beside me, which means I will make it. I love her for magically appearing: our eyes (hers, herb-garden hazel; mine, sky blue) lock and promise we'll work the shock out—and what it means for us—later. She and the nurse are iterating how "right" it was I came in. Though I "could have called an ambulance, you know." But I was just a mile away, I say. I don't mention that I knew where the emergency room was because six weeks earlier I had rushed to this hospital, Scripps Green, a half mile from the beach at La Jolla, when I was half-panicked, a chunk of silicone that I had buried in my ear canal for silence while sleeping was stuck. I'd had underwater hearing and couldn't think straight. The shock of the $350 bill came later, but the good doc tweezered the greasy lump out, then told me never to do such a dumb thing again. I also don't say that an hour earlier while hustling to my car I thought to drive home, a jet-fast three miles to get Suzanna and, with her, figure out what was wrong. This nurse would have admonished, "Had you done that, you probably wouldn't be alive."

These assessments keep interrupting what I want to be conscious of—blood draw; blood-pressure cuff; wristband; electronic chart; new faces, uniforms; dog-eyed gazes—and I sink back into myself where I need not participate, though I'm grateful they're reviving me, a rare spiritual tilt for me, primed as I am, as we all are, to put *this* moment off until the one day, *this* day, when mortality shuts our putting it off up.

What For • The nurse, vigilant at my worry, says, "You're getting emergency angioplasty very soon. Can you hold on?" I can. Suzanna kisses me, and I'm being rolled down the loud, slick hallways to the catheterization lab. (During my condition's onset, others snap-to with procedure; suddenly I'm their ward, agented, the gawk-dumb observer, my illness gathered round by far more people than I thought possible.) The wheeler asks about my pain, one to ten. "An eight," I say. But I also want to say I'm relieved, edging on giddy, to be alive *and* laid low, like a badly wounded soldier, pulled from combat and on a flight home, he believes, to recover. At least, he won't be by himself if he dies. *You're right, Mr. Larson. You're having a heart attack*. I'm surprised the attack is longer, not shorter. It's a nether-land I'm feet-dragging my way through now that the E.R. gang has stabilized me with a blood thinner, a clot buster, a diagnosis. I have time to stomach its yaw and gauge its slice, lifted onto the altar of *having* a heart attack and not yet having *had* one.

I'm the back-flat center of attention, fluorescent lights above me, film frames, clicking by, Ishmael adrift in Queequeg's coffin. The novel's ending reads, "I was he whom the Fates ordained." And then, "The unharming sharks, they glided by as if with padlocks on their mouths; the savage sea-hawks sailed with sheathed beaks." The orphan, abandoned and saved.

The smell of disinfectant and Ajax, the funhouse sound of wheels rubbering the floor, the creaky squeak of the bed's aluminum bars like wind-swayed chains—is it then that I look up, pausing at an electronic door and a passkey pinging it open, and regard again in Suzanna's frightened look the two women she carries—my tongue, she tells me later, curled out and onto my thin-lipped pucker with some talky intent: in that moment I recognize her double-sourced ache. First, for her grandson born three years ago with a chromosomal defect (lissencephaly) so severe that they fear he will not develop beyond infancy. Second, for her son, the boy's father, now forty-two, who, just after the boy arrived, was found to have tumors on his throat and spine, little black flags of cancer. On a bookshelf, Suzanna has posted their photos above a candle and incense base. There I have seen her pause—communing with the heaviness, the helplessness her grief begets.

And now she reaches down to palm my forehead, the heart patient who needs (*I'm sorry*) son and grandson to move over so he—so *I*—receive the anxiety and sorrow she renders them.

Unclogged • The cardiologist tells me to watch a monitor as he performs the angioplasty. (His card, which I consult later, reads "interventionist," a title reminiscent of a medical exorcist or a latter-day shaman.) I'm shaking like I'm freezing. I am freezing and frightened. "Don't worry," he says. "We've done this a thousand times." But, I think, not on me. Above my chest he glides the fluoroscope, a Cyclopean eye, projecting real-time images of my arteries. He clicks it on and there, on a screen, is my turbulence, X-rayed within. (All this high-tech jargon I cobble together weeks after.) He says, "I need you to pay attention. Hold your breath when I say so, OK?" OK. He tells me he's puncturing my groin for the catheter. *Punct*, and for a few hard moments I feel a hose inched in. He says that's done, and now the dye's coming. On the screen, my arteries darken and animate. "See them?" Yes, I do. Floating in some grey, groundless landscape, they are pulsing. They jump and jerk. Puppets on sticks. The broad, flat scope above me rotates, tilts, turns, pulls back, repositions, and hastens in close, robotic motion with spasmodic intent. I can't quite tell whether the image is gyrating, the cath line is wriggling, or the electrical voltage is causing it to shake. (Later, I download a YouTube angioplasty video that shows such quaking is actually the excited beating of a human heart. The flush of rescue.) "Hold your breath . . . and release." This is like vivisection:

live surgery. I see a squirming strand, like a car being chased, tracked by a night-vision camera, prodding its way through the artery's narrow passageway. "See the balloon?" Yes. It's an inflatable little barge, a cowcatcher sweeping away the debris. The balloon unplugs the artery. "Here comes the stent," he says. "Now hold your breath . . . and . . . and . . . release." I follow another tunneling in but already I'm feeling something other than breath release itself. Something like the light and the whoosh when a wrecking ball barrels open a building. That's my artery widened. That's my blood getting through. That's me, oxygenating. My body sighs; it need not work so damn hard. "Got it," the interventionist says. Meaning, he's placed the stent. (A stent is a pencil-lead-thin expandable wire mesh, made of a chromium alloy thirty-three millimeters long, three millimeters wide. Wedged in there for good.) "Two more to go." Two more? Holy shit! But it doesn't matter. He—*we've*—done this a thousand times, and now, include me. I feel revived. I'm back, on track and train. I know I'm back since I turn to see mortality's depot, its eternity of benches, its ticket-taker asleep. Where I was disembarked. And from which I am yanked back on board. "Got number two," he says. And I can hear the train whistle *woo-woo*, feel the wheels wobble, see the view blur.

Way, Way Up • I'm on a cloud, looking down at being attended to. The blue masks have left, the fluoroscope pulled up, the muted celebration begun. I've weathered the diciest part, and the moment is transcendent, Buddhistic. A man-on-the-mountaintop instant so towering that its godhead *ding* cannot last. Which is the point.

There's the nurse, who, memory says, is no-nonsense, pushing me on the post-op gurney into an extra-large elevator, no doubt the one I came up on. The space is large enough to fit patient, nurse-wheeler, family, priest/minister, a couple of doctors, plus the starting lineup of the 1964 St. Louis Cardinals. My head bounces, a love tap, as my driver runs me over the gap between the floor we're on and the elevator's purgatorial passage, a bump strong enough to slap me awake. I have survived the onslaught. A hellish three hours, initiated by panic and flight and topped off by the strangely contemplative stenting. (I wonder later, maybe all this was the morphine washing through me like a glass of Malbec, but then, I couldn't have been *that* stoned because I was conscious for the proceeding, especially during the stenting when I held my breath several times at the interventionist's command.) And yet getting on the elevator I'm in the beyond. Nested there, I blurt out to my nurse-pusher, "You know what?"

This, just as the great industrial elevator doors rumble closed behind us.

"What?" She asks with such aplomb, such delight in her voice—as though I have just stopped her on the street corner because I must tell her that in that burgundy dress, her waist black-belted tight, her face-cradling auburn hair looped behind her ears, she's as pretty as the Fourth of July. This grandest of moments is mine. I'm being wheeled to recovery. I'm being delivered to my last act—and my last act has met me more than halfway. I'm enthralled by this feral feeling, which, before it passes, I need to make sure someone else knows I can name it.

"What?" the nurse asks again, with a touch of conspiratorial laughter.

"I'm in Nirvana—" I say.

And she replies, "I'll bet you are."

A Good Deal • When Dr. J, the cardiologist who has overseen my cath-lab stenting, believes I'm out of danger, he finds Suzanna in the waiting room. She's been there an hour, maybe two, thumbing a magazine, staring, she tells me later, at a smudgy window on whose darkness the high-beam fluorescents multiply the glare. I imagine a TV drama when he enters: scrubs with high stakes—white surgical mask around his neck, blue cloth cap on his head.

"He'll be OK," Dr. J says, his grey-blue eyes meeting hers with hope and resignation, the surgeon's gaze. "He's out of danger."

"Oh, thank you—" Suzanna says.

"But you should know, his coronary was serious." He says the two arteries that cover the heart and circulate the majority of the body's blood were blocked. Completely.

Suzanna says Dr. J's word, *serious*, shocked her; she heard trouble in his voice.

"By serious," he continues, "I mean there was damage."

Dr. J says that during my heart attack, a certain patch of the heart muscle's four million cells was deprived of blood. Lacking its oxygen, that patch of muscle died.

"How much?" Suzanna asks. Her hand, no doubt, cups her mouth, her breath stills.

"A good deal."

A good deal.

(Later, I jot this phrase down, buoyed by its double meaning: The same "good deal" my heart's been hurt is the "good deal" I got by making it to the cath lab in time.)

"What happens?" she asks Dr. J. "I mean now."

"We monitor him, we treat him with drugs, and"—he pauses—"we hope the next time he's stricken he's as close to a hospital as he was tonight."

The next time.

It's just a matter of time.

That moment, whenever it occurred, when I think, *I get it*, I wonder, in the moment that follows, what exactly it is I *get*.

You realize, Suzanna reminds me, hand-wringing, a week later at home, that we can't pretend this heart attack will never happen again. I wonder out loud, is that what I did prior: I "pretended" the one I just had wouldn't happen? Did I know it was coming and I would deny it? Really, I have that much power?

But, she continues, if I don't want another one, we (again *we*!) must adopt a new diet, embrace exercise, work less stressed, welcome our mortality, which is hell-bent on welcoming us. Or else we stay put. Manage the second coming of another, heart attack #2. Stray not from our southern California coastal home, a five-minute ambulance ride to Scripps Green and its heart-reviving cardiology unit.

There it is—on top of the burden of her family (there's no pretending there), her concern is already greater than the good-and-saved surgical feeling I'm so thankful for. At the same time I fear that I, who has been *her* support, now will become her patient.

He'll Live • The long, lie-awake morning after my late-evening angioplasty, I'm in my recovery bay, one of a dozen or so fully equipped stations that post-op patients occupy, usually for a few days. My groin bruise is pond-like and purple and throbs when I move an inch. That afternoon, after being told I should get up, I hobble around the bed. I lie back down, quickly. One of my sons enters, guardedly. He chats a while, runs low on exclamations, and is gone. I sense he's too shocked to deal with his old man's sail, blown and tattered by the death gale. Suzanna arrives, and she and I—I/V-tied and tottery—shuffle along the U-shaped wing, glimpse the other half-comatose lugs like me. Am I that ugly—the mussed hair, the fallen face, the doddering creep? We do an around-and-back through the ward. Rest. And another. Holding the gown closed behind me, I'm cold. I want my bed, its crib-cradle. She says, one more walk. I say, no. I inch back to my sick bay's machine-guarded warmth, sequestration. Recovery is supine. Recovery is morbid, slow.

There, I'm nested away. Twice a day, the attending cardiologist rakes open my privacy curtain with a metallic slash, sticks the cold disk of his stethoscope on my back ("Sit up, please," he says), registers my thumping. A nurse, in hourly checkups, pulls the cloth enclosure more gingerly. Still, I hear the ticking of the hooks, scraping along the runnel. Suzanna two-finger parts the curtain as though opening a puppet stage from which I, the marionette, perk up, semi-eager to engage.

At night, I try to sleep beside the soundless stare of the red-eyed machines, which encircle me like cockpit controls. There's the sac-dripping I/V, hung high on a metal T with hooks for additional sacs below. There's my uncoiling the lines of its tube. There's my old-man hobble to the bathroom: groin; pressure; pain. There's the three a.m. struggle when I'm too sleepy (or Ambien-ed) to get to the toilet. So I don't. Instead, I reach for the plastic jug waiting upright on the nightstand, rearrange my carcass sideways to aim from my shriven member a righteous stream. I hope I'm turned enough to bull's-eye. The jug pools with orange-yellow urine, its blast of stink a skunk spray. The sweet pungency of peeing says that the drainage part of me is functioning as it has in the past, so I must be getting better—ready to go home, get back to work.

Three Stents: Count 'Em • "Man, you were huffing and puffing," says John, holding forth at the foot of my hospital bed, "going up that hill." John's a good friend—he's more than that: he's one of my favorites because for years he seems to have read every one of the dozens of long-form, cover features I've written for a local weekly paper. He loves to quote the pithiest lines of those subjects I've interviewed; he often brags on my prose, "What a great story that was!"

Now, he and two other friends, Bob and Marc, are gathered round, their hands on the sidebars of my bed, looking down, not unlike a coffin view. John's describing how weighed down I was two Sundays before when we walked, panting my way to the top of La Jolla's hill, Mount Soledad.

John bends over, hands on kneecaps, miming my fatigue.

"Tomcat, that's how you were," he says. "Gasping. I knew something was wrong. Your tongue was hanging out." He laughs.

I think, the warning was there. Pure and simple.

John noticed. I didn't. Or else I was so busy trying to breathe that I couldn't grok how unusual it was that, on the way up, I was so breathless.

John is six-four and a voluble presence. I treasure his laugh, its loud impropriety, its unabashed disturbance. Hearing that means I'm back in the fold of friendship. Soon I'll return to the helter-skelter cheekiness of our Friday morning breakfast club, a men's group, which, with five core members, has met a dozen years straight in one of San Diego's many beachfront hash-houses where we shovel in the cheese omelets and buttered toast and joke and rant, mostly about politics.

I notice my pals are a bit vexed, not knowing what to offer me.

So, I say, "Christ, I never saw it coming. And to think"—I tell the story and conclude that the hardest part that night was letting my students go without an assignment—"I needed to finish the class."

"Mr. Responsibility," says Marc.

There's something new: their collective mask—the saggy eyes, the cloister-y smiles. *This has entangled you and spared us—for now.*

"So how much hardware did they put in?"

"Three stents," I say. "Count 'em." Two in the right coronary artery and one in the left circumflex artery. "I was ninety-nine and one-hundred percent blocked."

All three men goggle me like dogs watching a card trick.

"Look—here's what I've been reading." I start quoting the heart's facts and its menacing coronary breakdown, culled from a pile of pamphlets that appeared on my beside table. The nurses? Suzanna?

Here's what I've learned:

Weighing a pound, the heart's the size of your fist. It generates sixty times more energy than any other organ in the body, beating 100,000 times a day, 36,500,000 times a year, 2,555,000,000 times over a seventy-year lifespan. Flawlessly, continuously ejecting 70 milliliters of blood into the aorta, each 70-milliliter shot traversing 100,000 kilometers of blood vessels, beating 70 times a minute and pumping 5 liters of blood every 60 seconds. The 432,000 liters of blood freight-training through everyone every day. Its four chambers—two atria and two ventricles—with the left and right atria on top of the left and right ventricles, are blood-filling cavities above expanding-and-contracting pumps. The body uses the blood, depletes it of its oxygen, and the lungs re-oxygenate the blood. The left ventricle pumps blood into every single-cell-wide capillary and up and down the inch-wide superior and inferior vena cava.

A heart attack begins in the coronary artery when an atheroma ruptures, blood platelets rush to the wound, a clot forms, and the artery's flow is partially or fully blocked. An atheroma (literally, gruel growth) is an arterial deposit, composed of lipids or cholesterol, debris, connective tissue, and calcium. This sludge, as it's called, lodges in the arterial wall and forms a kind of pimple, better known as a plaque. Over time, plaques harden the arterial walls, a condition called arteriosclerosis. Some caps take fifteen years to grow. These old, grayish-white plaques are seldom vulnerable, their covering thick with calcium. You might think of old plaques like your father's bowling trophies, rusting memories to another era. A vulnerable plaque is an opaque, yellowish-white patch covered by a fibrous cap. Newly formed, these plaques are burdened by blood turbulence, arterial pressure, or a fresh fusillade of tiny cholesterol pellets. One day they may burst. One day they do. Their thin cap fissures and ruptures. A burst plaque oozes gelatinous gruel into the passageway.

"And that's it," I say. "Just one plaque—just *one*—boom!" Which is what happened to me. The wall caved. But the balloon angioplasty squished the globules aside, and the stents scaffolded the arteries. The bottleneck opening. "I should be fine," I assure them. "Here—look at these."

From a folder, I pull out the before-and-after X-ray photos of my coronary arteries. In the first image, the main gray-white spidery veins are clogged up.

"This one is death," I say.

Next, the photo of my opened coronaries, stented, all lanes go, freshly paved, if not a Ferrari, then a Buick 6.

"And this one. Is life."

They pass the photos around unmockingly. Hearts entangled are never spared.

You Were Dying • On Friday when I leave the hospital I receive several parting gifts. Among them diet instructions, a follow-up appointment slip, three stent cards (containing type, serial number, and date of their placement), a small bottle of nitro tablets (nestled in my fanny pack), a list of prescription drugs I'll take "for life." Several brochures comprise my reading. One on coronary artery disease is published by Abbott Labs, the makers of my stents.

Sitting at my desk, with the Abbott info, I'm struck by this guileless line: "The first symptom of heart disease is sudden death." Meaning—had I died, I would have had none of the secondary symptoms, the indignant *Christ, not now*, the vicelike chest pain, the wedged-in-a-tunnel fear. I got through my heart attack, a dubious achievement, after which I'm awarded the nonrefundable prize, a heart condition. Thanks to the cath lab and the cardiologists, and my good fortune to be a mile from the hospital, I'm still kicking, albeit pinned between "it's here" and "now what?"

How happy can a man who's cheated death *be*?

Very happy, I decide. I'm returned to my sense of wonder, now more sharply teleological than ever. When you don't die, you get to be as philosophical about death as you like. The unanswerable, though welcome, questions queue. Is it possible to move before the bullet's impact? Halfway from the bridge to the water, does regret reverse the plunge? How much time *do* I have?

Such indirections initiate a new drama—the comedy of blood.

Reading on, I find another of the pamphlet's gems: "It is possible to have a heart attack without experiencing any symptoms." Then I remember what one of the cardiology team, who warmly gripped my hand in the recovery bay, told me.

"You were dying. Did you know that?"

I understood the statement and the question. I was thankful to hear him say *were*. But did I *know* I was dying? In what way might I have known it? I sensed my death may have been approaching. And I was worried I was dying. *That's* why I rushed in for help. But in the moment I was dying, no, I didn't know I was. I knew it only after the cardiologist told me. So it doesn't count, this (useless, self-contradictory) adage: sudden death will kill you. It's merely one of the disease's many devious ironies. Despite what those "sent back: he's not done with me yet" bestsellers say, I doubt there's an after-death—the euphemism is afterlife—where you wake up and say, I just had a heart attack that killed me. I doubt there's a heaven, or hell, or limbo, in which you or I are judged or carry on or waste away. There is only what we project or predict about our ends.

So no, I didn't know I was dying, in part, because we are, as long as we live, *not dying*. And when we do die, we can't know anything. It's over.

Imagining all that, it's no wonder I embrace those two defiant words. Not dying is the maintenance regime my heart has been on for years. Does it know any other? My heart has not been telling me my dying is coming. On the contrary. Only my *mind* tells me that. The heart is no Tiresias, burning a crow's entrails to dial in the future. If the organ has always tick-tocked, why would it stop or, just as bad, fake failure, warning me that it might cease beating? Is the heart capable of such subterfuge? (I mean medically, not metaphorically.) It works well or poorly, up-to-speed or snail-slow. It works until it doesn't. And, as a caution, I realize angina ushers in the fright of suffocation. Yet the pain passes, as does much of its remembrance. Otherwise, mothers—so I'm told—would never have another child.

In evolutionary terms, the passing of fear and pain prescribes our heedlessness. Running wild is the engine of youth. Experience teaches us we're often incapable of learning much from experience, though we fancy that what just happened is a great teacher. Another fatuous maxim. I've never understood this. Why are we so incorrigible with diet, romance, faith? One reason is, if we were wise before our time, we wouldn't enjoy lolling in the palm-shaded isles of art, myth, literature, and religion, what David Rieff calls "the consolation of unreason."

Not dying is like a guardian who stands sentry against an invader. If the invader never comes, the sentry issues no warning, and the community's startle reflex withers. If the invader does come, the overtaking is so swift—the tsunami, the quake, Little Boy falling on Hiroshima, Fat Man on Nagasaki—that our first reaction, to doubt the siren, is all we're really capable of.

The Clash Comes Home • Sunday morning I have a big mug of coffee and feel stomach-sick, panicky. I lie down, wrist on my forehead. I'm wired like I haven't been in weeks: I decide it's my wide-open arteries rushing caffeine to every cell. I'm so reamed out and blooded (medieval physiologists called it sanguinity, the complexion ruddy, the temperament optimistic, romantic) that I'm prey to more neuronal excitability than I've known.

So instead I drink green tea and settle down.

Some friends think I should be in bed. Hell with that.

Come afternoon, Suzanna and I walk. I put on my plaid-green Pendleton, with the quilt-stitched insulation, and my black sweatpants; she, in pink top/bottom sweats, her stay-at-homes. Onto the sidewalk we go. Years past, we walked to Starbucks with the Sunday newspaper. But that lapsed. Categorize this outing as doctor's orders.

Sandaled feet, I shuffle along, the sound of slippers scuffing the walkway. Suzanna grabs my hand, holds it for a few seconds, squeezes, lets it go. I go in and out of her care. I'm the child, guided on my bike, parental unit beside me. I want her guidance—and I don't want her fussing, this dependency and what it represents: a *me* I'm not about to be, one I must avoid.

We pass the crowded-together shoebox houses of our 1950s-era suburb. We pass the handiwork of homeowners, each domicile landscaped with drought-resistant bushes and Bird of Paradise plants. Their squawk-open beak-heads are existentially alert: the bright orange crown and soft blue tongue explode atop the dull green stalk. We pass one ugly two-story house after another, one where Mr. Multi-Equipped Homeowner parks his giant boats in the front yard, where every other October he posts signs for Republican candidates, the de facto party of San Diego, Navy Town.

Driving by those signs, I used to cringe, seeing the vile name, Duke Cunningham for Congress. Now, toddling through, such cares have fled.

We walk farther, head up a new block.

Suzanna says, "Can you get out—can *we* get out—like this, every afternoon?"

"Oh, honey, let's not plan it," I say.

"I know, but I'd like to set a time."

Once Suzanna and I rushed to the bedroom to have sex whenever we wanted. Clothed fucking I think we called it. Then one day we noticed we didn't do that as often. So we started, smart grownups, to schedule our liaisons: Monday, 5:00 p.m., sex. And it happened. Partnership's second half: calendar it.

"OK, you're right," I say. "I need this."

"We need this," she says.

"*We* need this," I agree.

Going on, silent, we float by the midday barrenness of the houses. And then, it occurs to me, that just by walking this neighborhood, its salutary effect is as much mine as anyone else's—the daily stroll of the cane-tapping Vietnamese man, in blue sweater and fedora, who sleeps in a house with midget trees, perfectly pruned, and to whom, as he passes us now, we slow, bow, and bid hello, one survivor to another.

The Heart's Will • How did I remain upright that Monday evening when two of my coronary arteries were all-at-once blocked? A neighbor, who's a nurse, comes over once I'm home and describes the body's blooded will. The adult heart is a muscle, and like any muscle needs fresh blood. The arteries, which hug the heart like a baby hooked on its mother's nipple, have branches or veins themselves that perforate the organ. When the coronary arteries are obstructed, the incoming and outgoing blood finds other ways to deliver its payload. It's called collateral flow.

Such flow is akin to how water moves in the Robert Bly poem, "Mourning Pablo Neruda." Water, Bly writes, "*doesn't care / about us;*

it goes / around us / . . . always closer / to where / it has to be." Collateralized veins river new pathways for the blood. These paths speak to our evolutionary longevity, our ongoingness. I'm fond of how Dr. Caldwell Esselstyn characterizes collateralization: "Coronary arteries actually perform their own bypasses."

Doctors know from autopsies that such new highways are common in the gummed-up passages of older people. Doctors also know that when young athletes die of cardiac arrest, collateralization has not occurred. Recall the college basketball star Hank Gathers, a twenty-one-year-old in the prime of his playing career who collapsed and died during a game in 1990. His autopsy revealed that his sudden arterial occlusion (one hundred percent) turned a vital heart from a rare-steak red to a bloodless yellow-brown in an instant. A plaque burst, and Gathers blacked out. He was gone almost as quickly as he hit the floor. Unlike him, older and better adapted, I had enough obstacle-avoiding flow to give me time to drive myself to the hospital. (Though now I know it is *not* recommended.)

What I find astounding (at the time, I make little sense of this in my journal or conversing with others) is that the angina (the guardrail) and the ensuing heart attack (the plunge down the ravine) transpired only when my coronary arteries had nearly shut down. My dairy-rich diet, my genes, a breath-sapping uphill hike, and my Monday evening trauma while teaching coalesced to choke off the blood supply. A calcite drip takes an eon to close a cave's opening. Collateral flow kept my heart muscle going, barely lighting its way. At the same time, collateral flow kept *me* in the dark so I didn't realize the buildup of plaque was, over my five-plus decades, irreversible.

The emphasis is on fate's fickleness: As your body is slowly killing you, it's just as defiantly keeping you alive. If life keeps death at bay, how are we to unveil the wanton subterfuge of a death-welcoming disease?

Approaching Epilogue • Dr. J says I can teach on Monday evening, one week after the event. If I feel up to it. I do. Suzanna drives me to class. And stays throughout—adamantly watching as I knee-bend to pick up dropped chalk, perking up as I air-out my lungs. To the group, who sit backbone straight, dazzled by my quick return, I apologize sheepishly. (Part of me feels I shouldn't be in class. Not that I don't deserve to be back—deserving or not means nothing: the odds were greater that as arterially thwarted as I was, I should have died.) One student asks if we'll make up the class they missed. He paid good money for these nine weeks of instruction, he says, with an embarrassed laugh. I ask the students if this is what they want. There's no enthusiasm. We'll see, I say. Before I spin my story, I ask them what they recall. They knew something bad had happened to me by the look of terror on my face—so much for the mask I thought I'd adopted—and I left so fast that they just looked at one another, flummoxed, and went home, glad for the break. My tale doesn't go into the hospital drama; instead, I focus on the medical miracle of stents.

Riding home, I realize how fast the night my heart drove old me down is over; this wounded hero now has his legacy. One week on and I can say I've *had* a heart attack. Odd that I'd feel some cachet with that phrase. And, the best news, I'm better. Dare I translate *better* into healing? I don't understand, but *better* feels both uncomplicated and messy.

I feel a tad lighter, probably lost ten pounds. Though I don't dare weigh myself. Why does it take a heart attack to get me below 220?

Two weeks out, I feel there's a newness to my place in the world. It's like I'm living in a space reserved for someone else. Familiar haunts *aha*: the hot air rising from a canyon, the briny smell of an ocean tide pool. I'm stirred by my senses in spaces I already know because I almost lost them: how much I'm trembling, the weather vane inside spinning, realizing what I would have missed had I died. Without me, what is the world? What's more, a world without me forestalled, my "I" is now profoundly singular. If possible, I'm more self-possessed than ever. This *not being dead* defines me. I'm my own replicant. Twinned as it were. The old me is back. He's newer and older.

One evening, Suzanna asks me to sit on our green couch in the front room and talk.

Right off, she admits that she's having a hard time with this.

"With what?"

"I'm worried about you."

I snort.

"I mean it. I'm worried that you're not paying attention to what's happened."

She says she believes I've already flopped back to past behaviors.

"No, wait a minute," I say. "I'm doing really well. I exercise. I've lost some weight. I'm calmer. What do I need to change?" I'm a bit heated.

She says that an illness means paying attention to oneself in a wholly new way. She compares it to one of those flashing yellow lights at an intersection. "You're being warned something is coming."

"What's coming?"

"Another heart attack."

"But I have stents," I say, turning on her, abruptly. "My arteries are open. I wouldn't be here now if they weren't. What more do you want me to do?" A siren-like urgency amps up my words.

"*That*," she says. "Get angry."

"I am angry."

"I want you to get angry *and* get busy. I want you to work out with James," her twice-weekly personal trainer—"go to Meyerhart," her naturopathic doctor—"get one of those heart-screen MRI tests"—"start cooking, work less, eat protein, take walks, get a massage." In short, I think, adopt *her* longevity program, a bit galling to me when she's not sick. (It's not lost on me that maybe that's why she's not.)

Then I remember. One cupboard bulges with white, fat, plastic jars of "Functional Food," "Vegan Protein Shake Mix," "Inflammatory Powder." There are barbells and dumbbells in the exercise room, a big green ball for stretching. There's a yoga schedule on a kitchen closet door. The house has begun rattling under the throes of a new Vitamix. She puts lists of recommendations on my desk. One is "Work to clear the Virgo sign of *victim*." (September birthday.) Another, from her oldest friend, a doctor's daughter in Louisville, Kentucky, reads: "dairy causes inflammation . . . plaque is attracted to inflammation in artery . . . arteriosclerosis is an inflammatory disease . . . read Dean Ornish . . . local doctor's food plan: no animal products . . . success with his patients . . . vegan plan reduces arterial diseases."

"But," I say, "I've been a vegetarian for twenty-five years."

Her look is less than quizzical.

To Suzanna, all I seem to want to do is sit on the couch and feel my blood flow because I'm appreciative of what it would have been like had I not been able to sit on the couch and feel my blood flow.

I ask her, "Don't you think I'm better off?"

"Yeah, I think you're better off. But—"

"But what?"

"But I want you to check out alternative approaches, see other doctors."

"I'm doing as much as I can," I say.

"I'm worried it's not enough."

"You know, I don't like where this is going," I say, standing up. "Talking like this at night is no good." I remind her how much I hate ending the day on a contentious note. Visions of my first marriage, especially its nasty end when such fights meant I slept on the couch. "We'll talk tomorrow," I say. "That's what tomorrow's for."

And with that she's up, heading for the stairs.

I stand, flat-footed. I should but I don't call her back. I'm being scolded, and after all I've been through? The indignity of a heart attack and then this: *her* pulling my responsibility to her out of me like a lung harvested for another's air.

Minutes later, she comes back down in her nightgown, hugs me and says, "I don't want to lose you. That's all."

Her eyes are gifts. I cannot *not* receive them.

A cardboard cutout, I hug back feebly.

She turns and again goes upstairs.

The faucet turns. Indeed, I am angry that I'm not allowed to savor the new time I got. She's already pushing to enlist my rivering bloodedness to fight invader and occupier. But I'm *not* strong yet at the broken place. I'm just trying to figure out what I'm up against, which is not helped by the nebulousness I feel.

Wasn't I fixed?

If so, how come I'm still ill?

I remember then that her grandson's and son's options are fewer than mine. Of their fate, I've been saved, or so I like to think. It's true: I'm the one who's less in need. The new fact, only half-conscious in our relationship and as such outweighing everything, is her mounting *number* of potential losses: son, grandson, me. Three male generations.

Emotionally, she's most in need.

I see that my condition has unmoored her upon an inconsolable sea she can no longer keep at bay.

But when I crawl into bed, cuddle and kiss the hair covering her neck, clasp her shoulders, cheek-touch and covet them as before, I realize what I want is to possess her body, its bow-like bend, arching back to me, taut and pinned, there still when we awaken.

For the Time Remaining • And yet, before dawn and down the waterslide of sleep, my storm-drenched phrase, *I'm sorry*, returns—words I had little hand, though much voice, in uttering. They seem truer than what I didn't say. Some flaky reassurance, like: *Don't worry, honey, I'll be all right.* A statement that, when it says, Don't bother about me, is a plea to be bothered about. Even—and especially—with sudden illness, the duplicity shines.

What I wanted to say I was sorry for is that I let you down. Had I stayed in shape, fasted the fat away, been mindful of my disease's inevitability, you would have my arms to enclose you.

I'm sorry that the flying net, its squares of roped air, landed on you.

I'm sorry that you'll outlive me.

You're sitting in our new home addition, the sunroom, staring through the floor-to-ceiling windows across the pool to the canyon's other side, its steep plunge, its patches of ice plant, the block-long park on the mesa above it where the eucalyptus trees, their insatiable verticality, drink up the sun—and I'm gone.

I'm sorry.

That when we're together and I'm adrift and you suspect I'm bored and not paying attention, I'm drawn to all those times I'm remembering you.

Your chestnut hair, sparkling in sunlight. (*Don't cut it short*, I tell you.) Your collages. Your stone-heavy rings. Your sentry eyes. Your quivering stomach (and my cheek there, kissing just above your foresty tuft). Your operatic orgasm. Its tremor, its evaporation. Your arms encircling my neck, your elevating toes, your lung-emptying *ump* when we embrace. Your chopping onions and greens and whistling "Way Down Upon the Suwannee River" in one key, which, midway through, you modulate to a key a halftone higher. Your Sunday phone calls to Ellen, your Louisville friend, intoning *we* more often than *I*. Your match-lit glow to greet me, mornings, in a skimpy red toga, setting the coffee down, and evenings, your whooping with impish delight that I've come home. (Once, and this I, also, regret, I scolded you for peppering me with questions the moment I came in, and would you mind waiting, at least, until I've dropped my bag and taken a leak? Your ardor squelched. Your injured surge. My malice still stings.) Your Epsom baths. Your Mongolian rugs. Your blue-jay blues, your crow-black blacks. Your admission in therapy when our Jungian analyst blurted out, "It's obvious that you love him."

"I do love him," you said.

It's obvious.

I'm sorry.

For the boy's birth defect, for your son's cancer.

For my heart disease.

For our lark-like life—our hovering, our turn.

For the timelessness of the time remaining.

TWO

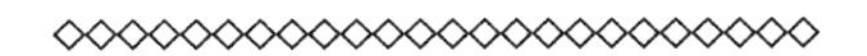

To articulate the past historically
does not mean to recognize it "the way it really was."
It means to seize hold of a memory as it flashes up
at a moment of danger.
— Walter Benjamin, "On the Concept of History"

Running in the Family • A month after my infarction (the clinical term we, the initiated, use), my niece, Akasha, arrives for a weeklong visit. She's the daughter of my older brother Steve, who died at forty-two, in April 1989, from, you guessed it—heart disease.

At nineteen, she's a big girl. Five ten. With Steve's big shoulders and wide girth. An open-faced Midwesterner. Her blue eyes are clear, uncorrupted, songs of the North. She and I have never talked before about hard things, and we turn our attention at once to her dad. Share photos. Then stories. She says she grew up "rough," as her stepbrother labeled her childhood—no electricity, no indoor toilet, just one woodstove to heat a rangy house during Wisconsin's arctic winters. Whatever was dished out. She learned to take it.

Akasha was less than two and has no memory of Steve's keeling over beside her crib. But, as family lore, she and her mother pieced together its mystery. I've added my two cents.

The year before he went, Steve had a recurring, radiating pain in his arms, back, and stomach. To deal with it, he'd get in his truck and drive the rural roads of northern Wisconsin where he and his wife lived. At the time, he was in his early forties, a high school teacher. When he told his doctor about his malady, the man diagnosed severe heartburn. This made sense to Steve. He was, by then, 280 pounds, sedentary, overworked, addicted to Wisconsin cheese. His wife said Steve dealt with the arm/neck pain, the stomachaches, by finding fault with her or her two small children, his stepsons. (Akasha had just been born in 1987.) Storming out, he'd climb in his Ford truck. For hours, he'd plow the highways. The truck's treads rolled, its heater baked. Every so often he'd stop to vomit or cry or cough it up. Nothing emerged. The pain, in chest or stomach, must have been excruciating. Steve would stop at a convenience store and buy Maalox—sip the chalky sauce, steel his roiling gut. What was this affliction? All he knew is that *he* had to endure it. And sure enough each flight from home and into the eruptive pain convinced him his truck cure worked. Especially since he came back to wife and kids purged, stabilized, the matter resolved.

Steve never told anyone of his drive-around drama. (How like collateral flow it is, Steve and his truck and the Maalox rerouting the problem he did/didn't know he had.) He never fessed up until he had his first mammoth heart attack in March 1989, for which he had an emergency triple bypass. It was then the cardiologists discovered the muscle of his heart, as he told me on the phone, "was half dead—and had been for five years." Half of the muscle had been deprived of oxygen and was useless. During Steve's bypass, the surgeons carved him open and found whitish scars, as well as dark areas of necrotic cells, that they espied through the pericardium, the wet fibrous sac that surrounds the heart. With three nearly blocked arteries, the tissue was blackly scarred. To treat him, they harvested the great saphenous vein from his leg and used it to bypass the impaired coronaries, reroute his circuitry like a new interstate, I-660, around a city, yet another type of collateral flow.

All these facts Steve uttered with a kind of pious abstraction as though it wasn't him but another poor sod etherized on the table. Part of his denial, perhaps. At first, he said the heart attack was mild. Then he admitted it was severe and he'd need time, maybe a long time, to get better. And then he confessed to his truck-running.

"You mean," I said to Steve, "all the time you thought it was heartburn?"

"I was sure of it," he said. "That's what my G.P. said. But it wasn't heartburn. It was angina." As chest or arm or neck or stomach aches, angina is the Iago of pain. It's what pushed him onto those two-lane blacktops. And yet, post-surgery, perhaps the morphine high unabated, he voiced little regret. "Hey," he said, "I feel fine. I'll be back teaching by the first of May," only six weeks away.

(How well I understand now. When the blood's flowing, of course we feel fine. We go back to how we've always felt: inextinguishably alive—not dying.)

The bypass saved him. But not his life. The damage was so bad that three weeks hence another infarct stilled his heart for good.

One week after my brother's death, I was bending over to get a wrench in a hardware store. I straightened up so fast I twisted my back. I fell to the floor, cried out, and then, frozen at a tilt, barely crawled home. The upshot was, I couldn't fly (chiropractor's order) to Wisconsin for Steve's memorial service. My mother and my younger brother went. I have always regretted that the injury kept me home and feel now, talking with Akasha, that I should make it up to her.

I say as much to her. "I'm sorry I couldn't make it to his memorial. I suppose you don't remember it?"

"No," she says. With her cellphone and college sweatshirt, Akasha seems a world apart from her dad's demise.

I have a tape recording of Steve's service. I received two copies and asked my mother whether she wanted one. "Heavens no," she said. "I'm afraid to listen to it." I don't bring the tape up to Akasha. Another time, I think. Not because she can't take it. She can. But I can't. Not yet anyway. The more I disinter my family's history, the more I feel ensnared in its net.

Cardiology Waiting Room Blues • In April, Suzanna and I buy gift certificates at Daily's, a heart-healthy restaurant, and we search the hospital to reward the folks, whose names we don't know, who helped me. "Please give this to the person who was on duty the evening of March 6. I know it was their job. But he/she saved my life."

In June, I arrive for my first stress test.

Right off, the waiting room strikes me—purgatory's nursery. On the tight-weave chairs a dozen of us heart patients sit, mid-afternoon. Three receptionists officiate from their cubbies. We check in, fill out a pill-intake intake form. I carry a list of questions. Nearby me is a man, post-op, in a wheelchair, his head slumped, his wife and son jabbering in Chinese. A guy in a neck brace reads *Fortune.* A married couple whispers. A woman knits. Another woman in dark glasses, Jackie Kennedyish. A silent couple, forcibly not speaking. In the ward from which the attendant will come, I imagine the smell of catheters, tubes stuck in flesh, the caustic stink of a draining infection under the scrub-brush sparkle of this cardiology wing, computers on wheeled platforms, the weight scales, the boxes of purple gloves, the plastic holders where my file goes on the outside of the door so Dr. J can, in seconds, scan the chart of whichever room, like rowed animal cages in a zoo, he enters. When I call cardiology, the message recited in the wait queue is that Scripps, one of two giant San Diego hospital chains, sees 55,000 heart patients a year. We are the patient population, personalities only to ourselves. Unfrightened. If we occlude here, we'll be saved.

The stats I'm reading in a brochure grab my eye. After the first heart attack, four in five don't have another. Getting stented or bypassed and sticking on a statin drug is largely why. But for the twenty percent who have another attack, the odds are less good. Fewer survive a second and a third ordeal, my father and brother cases in point. And yet, is this what we're thinking in the waiting room, that eventually we'll die of our affliction?

Hardly. The door to the ward and its examination rooms is propped open. A twenty-something nurse appears, calls a name, takes another in. Not to be judged. But, like coming to Jesus, to be saved. The efficiency stirs the expectation. The maniacally texting daughter, her serenely aging mother beside her, pops erect when Mom's name is called.

"Thomas Larson?"

My name, a question.

I walk on the treadmill for eight minutes, easily all I can take, then lie down so Gene, the technician, can ultrasound my heart. Gene says he's looking at the "motility" of my heart's four chamber walls. Motility is the ability of a muscle to move spontaneously and independently. Doctor's orders, he reminds me. He can't reveal much, but he does say, with a wink, that as far as he's concerned I passed the test. Dr. J will, once I'm ushered into the cubicle to wait for his door tap, give me "the whole scoop."

Gene's right. Dr. J says the stents are OK, my passageways are open, the pills are working. With the good news, my written-out questions lie like tree-dropped apples on verdant ground. Dr. J is done in seven minutes, a record, I figure.

Through the magazine-strewn room, I see, despite the late afternoon hour, that it's as packed as when I came in. All that seatedness yawns with arrested *motility*.

I head for the coffee cart outside the hospital entrance and my triumphant creamy latte. Waiting, I open the brochure again, stare at the stat: four of five don't have another heart attack. Marvelous odds. Yet I wonder what the odds are for one who has my genetic history. I'll look that up later. For now, I'll live with the eighty percent, especially considering the gustatory glory of that first sip of the latte—my mind, constellated, is effervescing, and I'm fairly jogging to my car so happy my heart is healthy once more.

A Psycho-Sexual History • Probing further, we learn from Akasha that because of Steve's obesity, because of his heart problems, because of his fleeing home whenever his gut started roiling with supposed indigestion, he could not perform in bed. He was impotent. Consequently, he had to masturbate in a tube so his wife could be artificially inseminated. This is how Akasha was born. She calls her conception "second hand."

I think that she and her parents lost the intimate making of a child as well as its memory.

Later I read my journal of the time following Steve's death. His wife told me then that Steve was ashamed of his impotence, a further reason he drove the night highways.

I start investigating websites and learn that obese men are twice as likely to be impotent as fit men. Add in coronary artery disease, with clogged blood flows, and impotence is certain.

Suddenly my disease is less *and* more personal. *Less* because as I read about genetic predispositions and the role of fat, I'm struck by the everydayness of heart disease, its ubiquity in our culture. I sense I'm joining the ranks of the heart-patient population, the treatable, the worried, the codependent. *More* because I realize that impotence may also be my history.

I suspect that when my niece and I look at each other, neither of us sees our independence from Steve. I'm glad when she leaves (she is too, I sense), so I stop mulling his duplicities.

By the Time We Get to Phoenix • A cliché is bad not because it's true but because it's overused. Same with doing what we already know how to do. Soon after the infarction, I'm at my desk, writing more intensely than ever. In the next nine months, I research/interview/immerse-myself in five long articles—one with an Indian doctor who owns dozens of small motels, another (fourteen thousand words) about the 1987 cold-case murder of an African American newspaper publisher, and another about those who do "dirty jobs," featuring a man who cleans more than a hundred portable toilets every day. (Rushing home, I almost vomit on my way to the shower.) Whenever I plan a day, it's always with an eye to how much time I get to write. I've been like this for seven years since I quit my tenured position at San Diego City College for journalism. The analytical/organizational structure of writing, the uncertain progress of the daily labor, is all I want to do. Suddenly, glory be, my first book has been accepted for publication—a book about the memoir and its memoirist. My literary cred begins to swell once I'm traveling and teaching with the book. I'm energized by talking about the form I love. Heart disease seems suddenly in the past.

That spring, for a month's vacation, Suzanna and I drive to Santa Fe, New Mexico, where we rent a house. (My ex-wife and I—she a weaver, I a musician—lived in the City Different during the 1970s and 1980s; our twin sons, who are almost thirty, were born there.) Across the bottom of southern California, we traverse those unsettled expanses, the worst, the desert east of Yuma, Arizona. (We sleep in Phoenix, drive to Santa Fe the next day.) That stretch of Interstate 8 is a moonscape of chaparral where violently dead mountains dizzy the horizon, an occasional gas-station ruin pocks a service road. For one hundred miles, there's no E.R., no H gracing this portal of cactus and sand.

I'm watching for those Hospital signs, which I've never watched for until now.

Beyond Yuma, I notice many (many?) rusted car hulls in the roadside ditch. Some rest on their sides or tops but most on all fours, angled to the highway. The skew suggests the driver veered off the asphalt, braking quickly, because he, not the car, was imperiled. And there he stopped, alone, seat-belted in. The headlamps lighted the sagebrush, and the man struggled like film noir at his collar to let the air in. Car after car zipped by until the Highway Patrol was called, who then flash-lighted the myocardial casualty, a salesman he was, half a tank left.

Here's how Suzanna and I deflect the image.

A Walter Mosley audiobook, predictable characters—Phoenix 257 miles.

We discuss her son who is on a new statin drug that's checking the cancer's growth—Phoenix 198 miles.

The friends we'll have dinner with in Santa Fe, their quirks and passions, once again in our orbit—Phoenix 145 miles.

Cruise-control at eighty-five in our year-old Honda Accord—Phoenix 68 miles.

Gas up in Goodyear. There's no tug in my chest, none I imagine, either.

Nonetheless, the tiny bottle of nitro tablets jostles in the cupholder between us, and an erect Phoenix skyline harbors the hazy distance, hospitals with cardio wards, soon, I'm sure.

"That's a whole lot of desert we drove through," Suzanna says. "You weren't worried, were you?"

Tied to the Body • Here's a tale—unremembered until the relentlessness of my reflecting on my condition snaps it back in place—I've never told anyone.

I'm fourteen.

I've grown up in a fat family—seen my brother bullied for his obesity (*Fatty, fatty, two by four*) and stop every day at Woolworth's for oil-bathed, freshly glazed donuts before catching the bus home (the later the ride, the fewer the tormentors); watched my father curse Steve for eating too fast while most nights Dad himself downs a Hershey's chocolate-sauce-covered mound of vanilla ice cream; smelled the cheesy heat of my mother's macaroni, the greasy aroma of Oscar Meyer bologna, the waxy edge peeled off, the mayonnaise spread on white bread—all of it, plus whole milk, fledged in the Land of Lard. I'm not like my brother who is as big as a barn and whom Dad derides. But I'm afraid I'll wake up one day as big as a barn, my waist puffing out like a vacuum bag, so embarrassed that I won't swim in front of girls; I lie with a towel around my neck, back-flat on the concrete. I eat just as my family does, pile high and devour whatever Mom serves like there's no tomorrow. When I dress for school and my pants' waist clasp won't snap, I feel a desperation. If I don't stop, I'll be a tub of Jell-o like Steve.

We have just moved to St. Louis, in the middle of February. I'm told to walk to school and register. On the way, I worry how I'll find new friends. But I'm momentarily safe: no one knows of my fat fam. It's the perfect opportunity to change course. The Beatles have just played *The Ed Sullivan Show*, and it's led me to buy a guitar, learn chords with an instruction book on my own. When I see the Liverpudlians, I embrace the economy of their bodies. I want that for myself. Sexed-up with stovepipe black pants and pointy-toed Italian boots. As if running from gig to gig works off the cheeseburgers. I decide a musician I'll become since a musician has no stomach paunch, no male breasts, no love handles.

But soon I recall that I've brought the Wisconsin pounds with me, and I feel sickened that I'll be like this, share my brother's fate, forever. I recall my nutty science teacher who wondered aloud in class one day whether stretching one's skin would reduce one's body's fat. I make a plan.

I buy a length of clothesline at a hardware store. I cut four-foot pieces—the cottony smell tickles my nose—and tie long lengths to the four posts of my bed. (I love it that my brothers and I have our own rooms, a move I figure, years later, my generous, self-sacrificing Dad changed jobs, states, and homes for.) I cinch each strand to its post with two half-hitches, a knot I've learned in Boy Scouts. I secure my ankles the same, then grab the upper ropes. I'm splayed on the bed, a martyr on the rack. The only problem is, my wrists must be tied so I'm fully stretched and can't move.

Doing this every night, I believe, will elongate my skin while I sleep and trim me down. Maybe if I can save myself, I'll be an inspiration to my brother and father, and they will change, too.

But how do I tie my wrists?

I loosen the knots and go downstairs where Mom and Dad are watching TV. They retire every night at 10:17 after the local news and the weather forecast.

I tell them what I'm doing is a required science experiment: How much does skin stretch?

Upstairs, Dad is tired, uninterested; he's off to bed. I produce the rope lengths for Mom. Who is baffled. Who, while I lash my feet to the bedposts, says, "Tommy, this is nuts. I'm not tying you to the bed. I don't care if it is for school. It's nuts." I ask her *please* tie my hands. Just this once. "It's nuts," she says again and shuts my door.

Nuts. Bonkers. Insane. My head pillowed, the words roll through like marbles on a movie theater floor. I agree, she's right. I might have flailed away with nightmares, awoken screaming, straining against the knots all night. I sleep as before, happy not to be roped in.

But this tie to an adolescent's self-deception is illuminating. What I thought, age fourteen, would metabolize away my fat confirms that heart disease was, like a Manchurian implant, gestating inside me even then. But what's really being confirmed is how much my unchecked weight nags. When I am fat, then or now—the fat sows fear. For the fat, like a poison, keeps producing what can kill me.

All Right Already • In Santa Fe, altitude seven-thousand feet, there's a lot less air than sea-level San Diego. I feel it. I'm sighing. A lot. Suzanna hears it, too, and asks, "Should we even have come?"

I tell myself, as we walk up the gentle incline of Canyon Road, that the sighs, besides re-oxygenating the blood and inflating the lungs, signal not trouble but gratitude. An Elgar of breath (against that Iago of pain). Since the source of worry has fled, I hope to enjoy my re-bellowing as long as I can. Breathe in. Breathe out. The circle is unbroken.

Soon, when we reach #550, the two-room adobe my ex and I rented thirty years ago, another sigh escapes on its own, a virulent moan—*uummhhhuumm*.

"Are you all right?" Suzanna says.

When I react, "Of course I'm all right," the tetchiness in my response surprises us both.

Later, nearing a favorite restaurant, El Farol, another groan, and before she says a thing, I strike: "I'm . . . all . . . right."

She stops. I stop. We stare at each other. The punishing separation of my three-beat phrase says, *turn off the nurturing*. (The lightbulb of memory flipped on. How my grandfather would swipe at his wife, "Woman, don't fuss!") It's not Suzanna's fault that my health needs ministering to.

She insists I set up an appointment with a local cardiologist.

"Because of my sighing?"

"No. To have an emergency contact—in Santa Fe."

"I can't have you interrogating me every time I expel a breath."

I hoof on, she follows.

From behind, she stops and I turn around. "Tom, either you're all right or you're not all right. These sounds you make are driving me crazy. If you need help, say so."

OK, I say. I'll go to a cardiologist and get a clean bill of health and be done with it.

I pick one off the Internet, a doctor whose waiting room houses several very large people. He's an unperturbed sort of doc, neither old nor young; his practice is small, a few cubbies is all. He talks to me (I'm on the table, Suzanna's in the corner chair, writing notes), takes my blood, listens to my lungs and heart, says things seem fine. "There's lots worse off than you," he says. "You're taking all six meds, yes?"

A few days later he phones to say my cholesterol numbers are within reason. I shouldn't worry.

I tell Suzanna, but her gladness is clipped. I know she believes she foisted this checkup on me. That her managing me—if it's even a problem—comes from her being assigned a new role.

In our casita, she makes a high-protein smoothie. I watch her, that sullen determination with which she shoves in the celery, the kale, the powder. How buoyant she can be, grabbing my shirt sleeve and pulling me toward her, one of her frequent wake-me-up demonstrations. How often she says, "Just talk to me." Some mornings she spends an hour and a half on the phone with her son or a childhood friend, tasks I don't do—precious mornings are to remove myself from contact with others and contact myself.

I know she wants a constant exchange between us. Its opposite, a compartmentalized, withdrawn partner, typified how my ex-wife and I were, the oblivion of the marriage's end. Suzanna's husband often abandoned her; a womanizer, he'd leave and return like a feral cat. We've spoken of our long-lasting despair over our marriages, vowing never again to lose ourselves by letting a partnership rot, wake up one day to patterns set in stone, immutable. For her the fear of conflict reigns almost as supreme as the fear of nursing a man's recalcitrance. Because of her husband's regular absence and her avoiding the knockdown drag-outs, she was a miserable missus for seventeen years.

In between bursts of the blender, I see that a green smoothie is how she materializes what she believes is best. Doing for me what I don't do for myself. Engaging *us*. After all, she partakes of the kale-enriched, wheat-grass-infused drink, too.

For today, the tennis match across the net of my/our heart disease has played out. It's naptime. I head to the bedroom, shut the door, and lie down—claiming the space before she can—one way I curtail our processing.

Letting it go so I can sleep.

November 11, 1975 • My father, who needs money to support his Florida retirement, is manning a booth, a school supplies convention, held in the hangar-like grand ballroom of St. Louis's Chase Park Plaza hotel. At lunch, he eats the chicken a la king too fast. He coughs, tries to shrug it off, excuses himself, takes the elevator to the room where his wife, my mother, is. He lies on the bed. The coughing accelerates. He hacks and hacks. Mom says, "My God, John, what is it?" He stops coughing and clutches his throat. He can't breathe. She grabs the phone. Dials 911. His body remembers five years before, the airless clime of Denver, Colorado, where one day, another convention, he also couldn't breathe. *That* terror sent him to the hospital: he got in bed and had his first heart attack. At mother's urging, January, 1970, I rushed home. I found him, lodged in his big black recliner. He had just turned the TV off. His face was paunchy yet hollow, regret-filled, defeated. His body seemed anemic, half-paralyzed. He looked as if the heart attack had electrocuted him—the substance of his flesh below its dark Bohemian surface (he was adopted; a Czech/Swedish parentage) charred by the jolt. On a month's leave from work, he watched daytime soap operas. Paisley pajamas. A purple satin robe like a mansion-bound yet grizzled Hugh Hefner. How incongruous. After Denver, he gave up smoking, walked a mile a day, ate ice milk, as though it were healthier than his beloved ice cream. He healed and continued hating work until he and Mom headed to Florida.

Now, the angina is back. *Dorothy, I can't—get any—air.* He grabs at the maple-leaf-patterned bedspread. His body flag-flaps.

The world, a storm-tossed ship, and he rolls off the bed. *I can't breathe—Call an ambulance—It's my heart.* Within a minute, red-faced, bloated, he's on the floor, flopping around as though he's gripping a live wire. Then it/he stops. Medics barrel in. Too late. Cardiac arrest. He's gone.

Three days later, my brothers (Steve older, Jeff younger) and I fly to Mom's home in Sarasota, Florida, for Dad's funeral. In the coffin, the mortician has perked up his face with a dark beige rouge. I study the edges around his scalp, admire the grey-white pallor of death. There's my real father, still aging, as I look him over one last time. Post-burial, at home, we watch Mother go into his closet, stroke his old Navy uniform, palm his watch and fraternity pin, drop onto her chair at the kitchen table—and then withdraw to dwell inside a glass globe where my brothers and I have no access.

She discounts her suffering, says she doesn't need us to stay. We have children and spouses to attend to—a bit of a dig, I think, but warranted since each of us moved several states away. I'm flung the farthest in California. Steve, Jeff, and I choose not to participate intergenerationally with our parents as they did, or had to, with theirs. One of the best things about us, I believe, is that we embrace our displacement. Something Mom could not do. We shook our collective heads when she got a job, age fifty-five, in a dress shop in Sarasota, for $3.30 an hour. Voted for Ronald Reagan. Desperate, lonely, she moved back to Middletown, Ohio, our home in the 1950s, the last cold, grey, post-industrial spot on earth we and our kids wanted to spend Christmas.

After all these spindrift years, of my having told friends of my father's heart-attack death (a tale I often recount since I've been so wounded), of its hollowing out my already hollowed-out mother, of her passive-aggressive isolation, of her succumbing, April, 1994, to a fast-metastasizing lung cancer and not expressing to my brother and me the ravages of the radiation and chemo, how much sadness and regret I have for her still.

And then, again, my father—all those years I distanced myself from his irritations, his inability to control, let alone, lose his weight, his rage at Steve's eating. From that distance, I also admired him for not shirking his responsibilities: to mother, to providing cozy rooms for my brothers and me, to his drudge in the Navy during the "good" war. His magnanimity teeter-tottered with his disappointments. Still, I'm afraid that while his disease is waking up in me, I'm being swamped by his gruff attitudes and his Willy-Loman worries. I cannot limp the limp of denial that crippled Steve.

Now that I have my father's condition, I can no longer push him away. He's in me. His bulk, his anger, his longing for the trim, disciplined self he wished he had, which includes, I admit, his distancing himself from his children (his children distancing themselves from him, as mine are doing) and which, I imagine, and perhaps he did, too, I would replicate for him. His legacy, to integrate, to understand.

It's funny, but just as the plaque has been broken apart and my arteries opened up, so, too, has my family's history of rarely dealing with our disease and its psychology been loosened from its truss. The blood of the present turmoil is oxygenating the past.

Stickier • One night, at dinner with two other couples in Santa Fe, the festive surroundings of The Shed, just off the Plaza, its purple and salmon-colored walls, roughly plastered, the drooping doorways, the hot, baked plates of green chile enchiladas, when the questioning begins.

Tell us what happened.

The story of my running from class, angina rising like an invading Persian army, driving myself to the E.R. And the pugnaciously ambivalent words: "You were dying. Did you know that?"

How are you now?

I'm fine. Fine. (Do I tell them that I struggled up the hilly Dorothy Stewart trail, not having said that to Suzanna, either?)

Really?

Yes. I mean it. (I feel fine. Why wouldn't I?)

How could you be? It's been only a few months.

No one believes me.

I thought you'd be changed.

How so?

You know, different, beat.

Maybe I am different. But I'm also as I was. Aren't I?

I feel safer when I marshal the medical facts: the drugs I'm taking are tiny minesweepers, cow-catching the cholesterol, filtering and thinning the blood. My three stents have reopened the culvert, its pocked surface pushed back. Best part, I *want* to be better; I want to eat the enchilada with just a tad of sour cream, and I do.

Though it's evening, the golden light above in the clerestory windows has not yet faded. The restaurant is packed. The place reverberates so the table talk volume keeps rising. Those waiting hover outside for forty-five minutes, and it's not even opera season/Indian Market yet.

How much damage was there?

Damage? This woman who keeps asking must have victims in her family or the ailment in her.

I'm not sure, I say. Some. Not a lot. Which is it? The doctor said the heart attack was *serious*. I seldom use his word. But I imagine he meant serious as nearness to death, not permanent damage. At times it feels like a heart attack is a crime my body, the child, committed, and I, the parent, don't want to take responsibility because it's the little cuss's fault.

Why is this so repercussive, so destabilizing? All this attention. An echo chamber of facts and feelings. It's not that I didn't ask for it. Friends have heard. Friends want to know. I can't stop people from saying, *So I heard you had a heart attack*. I am stuck between the truth of it I don't know and the explanatory equivocations I give as I go. Why not just say this? They'd understand.

Walking home in the cooling dark, I say to Suzanna, though I'm not ill, I seem to be *seen* as such.

"Tom," she says, hammering the issue again, "it's not like a broken finger that mends and you move on and forget about it."

"And because of that, I'm never healed. I'm ever ill. Marked."

Like the war veteran, the freed hostage, the politician caught masturbating. How can I be shaped so totally by one event? What do the children of parents who lost home and hearth during the Great Depression say? "After Daddy sold the family radio—the one thing in the house that brought us pleasure—he was never the same. Never."

But aren't we more than our generational stamp, more than the blot of an incident? Of course we are. But that's not how we're seen. The public me is the one who fell. Though I don't see myself as twisted-up in my scant celebrity, I am. I'm *representative*.

Every year 1.1 million Americans have a heart attack. Four in five infarcts come out of nowhere; they're asymptomatic. Every year half of all heart attacks are fatal, killing half a million; one-third of them are under sixty-five. Many develop cardiovascular disease as they age: as I write, eighty-one million have high blood pressure; eighteen million have coronary artery disease (CAD, my cross-to-bear); seven million are suffering the complications of a stroke; another seven million the fatigue of heart failure—in all, one in three Americans die of cardiovascular illness, one of two adults.

As much as I don't see myself as a member of this club no one wants to join, I'm in. I'm one of the 1.1 million. I am *he*, the guy who's had a serious heart attack. The man with the glass eye who sees the doubletakes others see in him. Plus, I'm one of the eighteen million with CAD, who are more prone to suffer a stroke or have another attack than those who haven't been laid low.

What all this may turn into, if I'm not careful, is that I start playing the infarct card. I'm not special—but oh yes I am. Feel for me. I'm possessed. My meandering career includes those of felicitous musician, failed composer, college teacher, now midlife writer.

Throughout, I've had no omniscient caller brand me with a condition as this disfigurement has. Such certainty of self has always eluded me—and now, bidden and not, it's here.

Speaking of Water • Three decades ago, when my ex-wife and I were renting a casita on Canyon Road, we feuded constantly. We never slugged each other, but we came close. I blamed her for making a lot of money as a tourist-targeting weaver (sums she deemed hers, which meant her keeping tallies of what I owed: $5 for half of the gasoline, $3 for half of the restaurant tip; the bill for my marriage grew to thousands). She blamed me for earning only tips as a musician. For years I played guitar for restaurant patrons throughout town, a nightly noisy recital I grew to hate. I went into debt to go to university and study music composition. Exasperated with shouting matches (this worsens while we're tending toddlers), I'd leave to sit on a boulder down by the Santa Fe river, watch the water roil or trickle, depending on the season. Not unlike my brother Steve used to do in his truck.

Today, I'm beside the river again. The little stream has a robust snow melt; it's bullyingly loud.

What a difference! In the past, I'd sit and feel sorry for myself, plot my way out of the marriage, calculate how much money I'd need as a *single* father. At present, I feel much the opposite. Suzanna and I are not entering an Ice Age in which our problems pool and freeze.

So why am I out here?

It's habit. The water, manic though directed, provides the semblance of change—nothing says this water is any different than it was thirty years before. The pattern-play of the water that was then is now.

It's in the grace of habit that insight grows.

The stress of this condition is unlike the stress of my long-ago marriage to a woman with whom I was sound asleep, for whom I had the nagging wish that she revert to the person I had imagined she'd be, while she had the same longing that I'd revert as well. I'm thankful all that is evaporating.

Yet I can feel the tears of rage well up, the cage I got locked in (locked myself in) with and without her, whose bars I continue to rattle—*this* is what the water is rushing at: I'm still grieving the waste of those years. All that time she and I wasted being ill-suited—faking concern, faking compliance, hating ourselves for the fakery.

What's surprising, in the water's broadening roar, the cottonwood's scent, is that after the heart attack, I felt my health would be restored, and not these regrets, like marching skeletons, disinterring my marriage. Having gained time, why use any of it to rehearse *that* signature failure of my youth, whose book I seem never able to close? That's why I'm streamside, the moment commanding me to go back.

In the water, its falls and foams, is my mortality—its pools pausing and deepening before me, before overfilling and driving on to where it has to be. The slap-faced sting of death allows me to integrate my parents' fate with mine, my relational myopia for my ex with Suzanna. And, at last, be done with it.

Co-Casualties • In San Diego, late summer, months after the heart attack. The fog-abandoned blue heat of August beckons, bleaches, unfetters. I'm forgetting. I'm adapting. I'm healing. I'm moving on. I decide it's time Suzanna hears a tale I've been saving for her, about my mother.

At dinner, I say I want to tell her a story.

After our boys were born, Mom used to fly to Santa Fe to visit. She'd bring matching sweaters, baubled/bangled/needlepointed

Christmas stockings. The clothes were about as far as she went in mothering the twins. She even refrained from offering advice. (I told her I'd read Dr. Spock: "You know more than you think you do.") She slept on a rollaway bed in my home office, and we spent evenings sitting in the living room while the kids, kneeling on the floor, created spaceships out of Legos.

Once, after dinner, she mentioned that Dad, who had died three years earlier, had a premonition about his end. Postretirement, she said he nursed a fanatical goal: get to Sarasota and move into their new home. From St. Louis, he drove them to Florida in two days and worked madly on the place. Laying stepping stones to the garbage cans. Carpeting the back porch. Finalizing escrow and the mortgage. Ten chore-huffing days without a break, and Mother, one steamy morning, asked him to go to the beach. Since their arrival, they had not had a moment's fun. What sort of retirement was this anyway? she teased. Dad said he would rather take a nap than sit in the sand. He wasn't ready to relax; they'd have years to relax. Mother, miffed, said, "OK, I'll go by myself." She did, an act of self-determination, a rarity for her. She drove to the coast, parked, sulked, and waited past pride.

The moment she returned, he rushed at her: "I can't believe you'd leave me like that."

She remembered he was "visibly shaken. He didn't look good." His need to get *her* settled in their new digs was his way of preparing them for . . . . She misted over, telling my wife and me, "I believe I brought his coronary on that much sooner."

"Mother," I shook my head. "Dad had heart disease. It was inevitable. You're not responsible." To which her pleadingly blue eyes, gazing at our twin boys, said she was.

Across the kitchen table, our salads half-finished, the vinegary tang stinging the air, I ask Suzanna what she thinks of my recollection.

She's unsure. "Why are you telling me all this?"

Because, I say, "My mother shared my dad's and my brother's heart disease. They lived on in her. I think about that visit a lot now. I didn't know it then, but I started to change my attitude toward her." I pause, fork-push the thick-cut carrots to the side. "She had no choice. Marriage. Children. Stuck with Steve." Surprise, but I'm quivering a bit. "The point is," I exhale loudly, "before my heart attack, I saw her one way. On the sidelines. Now, I see her differently. I feel less of my father's and my brother's loss. Instead, I'm feeling her loss. The one who survives." I often don't speak like this, my words emotion-rich. "My mother just couldn't win. That's what I'm saying. The men were sick and then the men were dead and then she was sick—from the strain of having cared for them."

"I see," Suzanna says. "You want me to stop worrying. Is that it? Just like that? Stop worrying?"

She casts me that *look*, a judgmental burn.

I can tell I've exposed a nerve. In us both. I've already linked me to my father, now I'm tagging her to my mother's mode, or, at least, the way my mother cradled her loss of my father and my brother.

"*Suzanna*, I'm saying just the opposite. I want you to care for me. But don't you think that by caring for me you'll suffer the guilt my mother did?"

"No," she says, dropping, not throwing, her fork at the bowl. "I'm not going to be pulled into some pattern you have with your parents." The stare is intense, a mirrored sun.

I realize nothing good comes of comparing mother and lover. Suzanna adamantly rejects it. We have moved on from our marriage patterns or, at least, we're hyperconscious of the threat they pose. The same should apply to our parents' patterns. But like ants those patterns keep sneaking back in to feast on the smallest remnant of food either of us leaves out.

I love Suzanna's boundaries, borne of years of personal therapy to resolve (her word) an epidemic of long-ago family illnesses and conditions: her mother's depression and disapproval; her biological father's abandonment; her stepfather's scorn and rage; her ex-husband, once a stumblebum, now vanished and forgotten. While I have not erected such walls, I push my ex-wife and my mother into our dynamic so Suzanna must reject them.

"The stage and the play," I say, my fork resting in my bowl, "just get bigger and bigger."

"What do you mean?"

"My mother is the caretaker. And that role devolves to you. That's all. I mean, wouldn't you feel the kind of guilt she felt after my father died? That is, after I'm gone?"

Suzanna gets up, takes our plates to the sink. Reminds me it's my dish night. Places very light arms, like sweater sleeves, on my shoulders. Pulls back to regard me with that shifty stare, her eyes popping from one eye of mine to the other.

"I understand why you keep telling me about her," she says. "You think I don't have any choice when it comes to your condition. That you'll leave me—just like your mother was left."

This is crushingly clear.

"That's it exactly," I say.

"I don't know how I'll react when you're gone. All I know is I don't want it." She grabs me, pulls back, sees me eagerly waiting, hugs me again, and says, "I'll succumb to something—but it won't be that I caused your death."

"I know that," I say. "Still, it's good to hear."

"It's just—" and then she stifles a cry, but I clutch her heartily. I start swaying slowly, and she catches my rhythm. I want the moment to end this day and night. I sense we're united but in a way different from that saddest of tragicomedies, *Two for the Road*, with Albert Finney and Audrey Hepburn. We're trying not to be hostages to the past, as the story forces the film's characters to be. The takeaway is, Finney and Hepburn can *never* escape their history. The film sentences their fate. It's hard not to fall for such mythologies, which, unless Suzanna and I outfox them, will strangle us with or without the knots of heart disease.

Pasadena R&R • To celebrate my birthday in September (having made it *to* my birthday), Suzanna and I spend a long weekend in Pasadena: the Huntington Library (autographed manuscripts under very dim light), the Norton Simon art museum (a few Kandinskys I love), dinners *al fresco* on Colorado Boulevard (angel hair pasta, lots of bread and olive oil), a pair of shiatsu massages (a tiny Japanese woman, no English, who uses her knees to crawl over and soften up my back).

After stirring the pot of the past with Akasha about Steve, I'm eager Suzanna and I retrieve our lovemaking, robustly licentious until this year. At least that's how I remember our Oscar-worthy orgasms. Another reason to leave town for an expensive hotel suite. I always get what I ask for on my birthday.

Still, having heard about the impotence trials of my brother from my niece, I'm nervous that my brooding on his performance will spoil the deed.

Post-pasta, post-Malbec, we come back to the main floor elevator. Beside it, pinned to the wall by a strap, we note a defibrillator. Recently, we saw a defib at a local hotel in San Diego, donated by a friend of ours whose husband had a heart attack there, on the dance floor during his daughter's wedding, and died. He could have been saved by the device.

I take Viagra. (My physician has given me a sample pack.) First time. I don't tell Suzanna. I want to see what happens.

I'm soon hard, the intensity, dizzying. Dry mouth. Flush face. Crimson glow. Viagra is like a stent for the penis. Thankfully, it doesn't constrict my breathing. I just get stovetop hot.

Teased, I sit spread-eagle on the couch in our suite like some African king on his throne.

The thrumming, throbbing, tumescent aliveness, licked into submission—it doesn't take long.

To my pill, Suzie has her wand. Back-flat, her shouts echoing off the popcorn-covered ceiling, I'm on her breast like a baby, and her hoopla is as raucous as the Kentucky Derby.

Afterwards, I confess.

"Really? You felt you needed that?" she says, her face softened in that after-coitus glow. "You never used to—feel that way."

I do now, I say. I wanted to make sure I was stiff, make sure our animal furor returned. It's not the source of our love, but it's a major expression. Wondrous that our wildness (afterwards, I mock-apologize for saying all those dirty things) is a source of stability for us.

But here's the other rub. One is sexual or one is impotent *with* another.

While I'm thanking my cardiologists for the stents, I should be thanking Pfizer for Viagra. While I'm thanking my partner for attending to my heart disease, I should also be thanking her for attending to our thirty minutes of sordid bliss.

Dallying on the couch, watching Keith Olbermann, who is yammering agreeably on TV but yammering nonetheless, I'm feeling numb and scrunchy, plateaued after my Viagra ascent into a mountain meadow. I get up and lean over Suzanna, snoring away under the ultra-clean Hyatt bedsheets. I pass my splayed fingers through her thick auburn hair, through the self-applied streaks of blonde, that two-tone thing she does, which I adore. I can be myself. I need not fear anginal agony every time I steam with lust. Odd that I wasn't fearing such coronary distress before Viagra. Now *this* med returns my youth. Yet it also corrals and unleashes a new set of expectations. Because of the drugs and cardiology's bigheartedness, *we get the life we would not have had.*

Beautiful burden that.

The Cunning Art • In our culture, there are many expressions of heart disease and its most dramatic moment—the chest-clutching, pavement-falling, life-altering heart attack, which, in the depictions, a man (seldom a woman) suffers in public and, most often, just in time to be saved. There are medical and metaphoric languages to express it, there are cultural artifacts to represent it, and there are psychological interpretations to process it. There is as much fiction in the retelling of an individual's myocardial infarction as there is in the artist's refashioning it. Of the latter, the most common example is the "family" heart attack, the one whose shockwaves shape the sufferer's kin, friends, and loved ones more than him. Not surprisingly, Hollywood seems to have drawn these traumas out as morality plays, making women co-responsible and making men their dependents. I begin with the 1941 film of Lillian Hellman's play *The Little Foxes*.

Regina Giddens is the wife of Horace Giddens, who is tormented by her and his failing heart. Regina, played by Bette Davis, wants to hasten the acquisition of his fortune so, with his money, she can finance her and her daughter's escape from the small-town Alabama aristocracy of the early 1900s. Horace, played by Herbert Marshall, has been beaten down; he's confined to a wheelchair, and he sulks, albeit nobly. Marshall enacts his suffering with palpable discomfort—the sick man's labored walk and breathing, his eye-darting dread, his feverish swallow of a spoonful of medicine, perhaps liquid nitro, followed by only temporary relief. (In all scenes Marshall appears, he's in pain, and I can't take my eyes off him.) Davis badgers him viciously. Most appalling is how she feasts on his ailment: the closer he gets to death, the more she schemes to bring it about. Indeed, *heartlessness* defines them both: Marshall's weakening heart will stop, and Davis's heart is nonexistent. This clash speeds the drama (only the daughter and a few black servants care about him), suggesting that certain families then favored cruelty over compassion. With no bypass surgery or stenting, people avoided acknowledging a middle-aged man's illness. Plus, succumbing to heart disease was rarely forestalled. Embracing his fate, Marshall tells his wife he'll soon be dead. To which, she replies, she hopes it's sooner than later.

The heart-attack scene, directed by William Wyler, is a finely wrought contrast between her callous refusal to help him and his incapacitation. The viper Davis is reminding Marshall of her post-marriage disgust for him: "I thought you were such a soft, weak fool. You were so kind and understanding I didn't want you near me." Suddenly Marshall has a breathless moment. He starts sweating. He claws at his throat. He shudders as he's hit—the occlusion, the clot. Weakened, he wheels forward in his chair and pours a spoonful of nitro. He shakes, drops the bottle and spoon, and orders Davis to get his other bottle. She sits, a head-lighted deer, and does nothing. Marshall struggles to his feet and for the next minute, while Bette Davis stares unblinkingly, her gaze arrested on hope and terror, he stumbles past and behind her, behind her camera-facing stare, from couch to wall to foyer to staircase, and the medicine upstairs. He gets halfway up before collapsing. Only then does Davis blink and call the servants.

The death scene is much less histrionic. Tenderness takes over. We watch him hold his daughter's hand and kiss it, we see his last breath register on her face, and we notice her expression slip from the gratitude of his kiss to the shock of his departure. The father dies of his heart condition, and the daughter's heart is broken. And with it the story takes a twist: the daughter abandons her mother because her role in conniving Marshall's death, which Davis cannot wipe from her face, is suddenly evident to the daughter as well.

Via Marshall's performance (Davis won an Oscar, he did not), the scene blueprints how we think the heart patient goes. Or is supposed to go. Heart attacks provide us a dramatic exit. What's more, those who suffer the long fall do so morally. Mortality ennobles us. As we die, we expose the family's lies.

Though we rarely reach such justice in our final hour, the culture insists we reach it in art. Oh, how righteously the novels, the plays, and the movies spell it out. Art says we have not died untidy deaths, though most of us will. Art prepares our loved ones to make amends, arrive in time, confront the patriarch, establish succession, and achieve closure, though such ennobling seldom occurs. Art insists we make less messy that which is messier than we imagine or can handle. Indeed, we die as we think we have lived—art reshaping our incapacities as aesthetic understanding, art giving us meaning when in our time meaning is seldom found, art depicting trauma and loss as more lifelike than life itself so we believe what should have happened to us actually did, when it never did.

The Widowmaker • Two years out—my book about reading and writing memoir is successful; I'm teaching with it throughout the country; my weight settles, stays above 210; and my heart ailment lies dormant, though at times I sense a flare-up is imminent and then it doesn't flare up and I don't know what to think so I try to quit overthinking it, forget about it, replaced by this, my utterly porous new normal—until one Friday afternoon I'm about to interview a local AM celebrity for a feature story on the demise of local radio, a man to whom I extend a hand at Starbucks and from whom I expect a chip shot in his throaty baritone but instead get a weak shake and a glum face.

"Did you hear? Tim Russert just died of a massive heart attack."

I breathe in so fast my lungs convulse, like a pulled drain plug.

And that word—*massive*—meaning there was no stopping it. Death by avalanche. Russert is me. Russert *was* me.

"Are you all right?" the man asks.

My hand goes to my chest. Where? In his office. How? Heart disease, apparently. Why? There is no why. More queries only ricochet off the void.

At home, I tell Suzanna the news. She remembers him, the TV reporter, longtime host of *Meet the Press*.

"What's so disturbing," I say, "is I just watched him the other day. Questioning somebody. He seemed fine. He was such a passionate newsman."

I'm glued to the TV—the story is covered relentlessly—hand-wrung by scores of colleagues—Russert, beloved like Walter Cronkite and Peter Jennings were—the old-style reporter, beyond reproach—his interviews, always objective—opinions, never intrusive—the man, his colleagues say, *did* his homework (He did? Why then did he die?)—asked informed questions—probed, parried, objected—Democrats and Republicans found him formidable—epitomizing fairness. Why would such a reasonable man just keel over?

Over several days, the facts are unearthed. Russert's left anterior descending artery (LAD) was blocked. Completely. Such sudden death epitomizes cardiac arrest, especially in men; hence, the artery's nickname, the widowmaker. His autopsy shows an occlusion so abrupt and ischemia (the heart straining for blood) so great that he was gone in an instant. Russert had diabetes, an enlarged heart, and abdominal obesity. His heart condition was asymptomatic. He took a daily aspirin. His blood pressure, his doctor said, was high but "well-controlled." His bad cholesterol, LDL, was quite low, 68 mg. Two months ago, he performed well on a stress echocardiogram, though the test would not have caught a plaque about to burst. He had exercised on a treadmill that morning. That afternoon a plaque in his LAD ruptured, the wound inflamed, the passageway narrowed, spasmed, and swelled, the blood flow to his heart muscle slowed to a trickle and, within a minute, stopped. Russert's heart lost its oxygen. As a result, it beat wildly, irregularly—fibrillation, it's called. He collapsed and writhed on the floor. Then, without blood nourishing the brain, he went unconscious. For a few minutes a coworker applied CPR, while paramedics were called. Arriving quickly, they saw he was glassy-eyed and unresponsive. They defibrillated the heart three times—to defibrillate is to stop the unsynchronized contraction of muscle fibers, realign those fibers so the heart beats in sync again. The window for reviving a fibrillating heart is about five minutes. The estimate is, Russert was gone in four.

Here's the shocker for me: someone on TV says that only five percent who have a symptomless heart attack survive. He/she doesn't say, *ninety-five percent die*, but that's how I compute it. Still, I'm lucky. I had symptoms: muscle weakness and fatigue days prior; a day of angina; moments of profuse sweating. Did Russert have any of these symptoms *and* not tell anyone? The only way he may have upped his chances for surviving—in so far as he realized the risk and was having discomfort—was to bunk in the cath lab or sleep in a van parked near the emergency room.

Was there a way I knew what was coming? Should I have bunked in the cath lab? No. But write it so it doesn't sound like cozy invention, the memoirist's deft hand. There was a siren that night while I was teaching, a wailing on the order of the Fukushima nuclear plant during the tsunami telling me to flee for the hospital.

By the time the streams of commercials return and a screen shows Russert's photo and dates, 1950-2008, one last time, I turn the TV off, ponder in the dark. Part of me wishes I could feel as lousy as I feel. But I don't: my language-dominating security team won't let that happen.

I mentally combo the Larson male line (father and brother and sons—the latter, feral and independent and often incommunicative), my back-and-forth with Suzanna, and my mother's dread living on inside me, until I suspect such ordering sounds like a good story. My illness as a memoir, though I'm not ready to start writing it. No wonder I love the form. It has my back. The story, ever unfinished, will take me where I would not have gone without it. How Russert-like: the heartlessness of such a demise and its unknown timetable ensure its suspense.

Dead Man Stalking • The *New York Times* weighs in: "If there is any lesson in [Russert's] death, his doctors said, it is a reminder that heart disease can be silent, and that people, especially those with known risk factors, should pay attention to diet, blood pressure, weight and exercise—even if they are feeling fine."

Two years plus, and I guess I'm feeling fine. The argument, however, is that when feeling fine one must adopt a Herculean attentiveness to one's diet, blood pressure, weight, exercise. Or else one is not healing. My poundage fluctuates, but it remains too high, too close to Tim's. OK. But it's less of a concern since, un-Russert-like, I received (albeit just that once) the anginal warning, the one blaring kindness the sickle-carrying, heel-close, black-robe offers.

I review WebMD. Angina comes on as any combination of lightheadedness, dizziness, fatigue, shortness of breath, indigestion, and chest pain. It's constrictive and heavy, the three-hundred-pound sumo wrestler sitting on your chest, an ache that pulses and radiates—the roller-coaster wobble and dive is the worst—in your neck, shoulders, arms, throat, or jaw.

Pain worried away is labeled stable angina. If there's no response to rest, it's unstable, a true emergency. The stable kind, like a child's nightmare, can be soothed away. The unstable kind shrieks for help.

That said, there's a DMZ where angina roams, appearing actual and feigned. Where psychological and physical symptoms cohabit. Who believes you're having a heart attack if you've never had one? You're disinclined yourself to think it's the Big One if you've endured chest tightness and stomach indigestion other times in the past—*and, after rest, such symptoms have left.* So what if you ate the whole pizza, finished off the angel food cake. You've got a nasty case of heartburn. Even *that* word is misleading: the heart is not burning, the esophagus is, that foul, burped smell of stomach acid. (The Maximum Strength Pepcid AC package states: "Heartburn with lightheadedness, sweating, or dizziness may not be heartburn. It may be a sign of a more serious condition." Nicely vague, isn't it?)

The burning reason is that the esophagus curls around the trachea *and* touches the aorta. (Nature bundles our core.) Either angina is agitating the aorta and infecting the esophagus/trachea, or reflux is annoying the aorta and portending heart trouble. Differentiate them, if you can. Misdiagnosing angina as heartburn can be fatal. The key turn: with reflux, there's no sweating; with angina, there's sweating.

Didn't Russert sweat? Didn't he have a moment when he thought it odd that he was all of a sudden hot and wet and way past his morning workout?

Did he turn and say, to anyone, "My God, something's wrong with me?" Was he so enthralled by work that the moment he fell and began blacking out he missed realizing *this is my death*? Surely, that's given to us. In some shape. In some form. Surely.

THREE

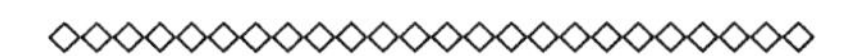

You meet your destiny on the road you take to avoid it.

—Carl Jung

I'm Not OK • Three days after Barack Obama is elected president, I give two lectures: one, on Friday afternoon, about his memoir, *Dreams from My Father*, another, in the evening (following a diet Coke and a veggie Panini with provolone), about the rise and swagger of this self-disclosing form—two talks a prelude to a Saturday workshop with twenty-five memoirists in Lancaster, Pennsylvania.

Near eleven, Suzanna and I return to our hotel room. She gets in her nightgown, I, in my red T-shirt. On Ambien, we're soon asleep in a bed way bigger than us, open suitcases on chairs, the room gold-gilt and carpet-cushy.

Snapped awake, I see the digital clock's red numbers, 4:11. Sweat's clinging to my shirt, forced hot air from a ceiling grill smells of baked dust.

Up, in the bathroom, on the toilet. The shower rug folded on the tub's edge. A chapel-like silence. *As you were* chimes in my mind. How long's it been? I'm trying to extrude a hot muck from chest and shoulders. The lava's stuck.

In the background, the faint heave and buzz of Suzanna's breathing animals the shadow dark, another-world species I hear as balm.

Back to bed. The red-faced numbers have gained a few. No real momentum. The forced-air blower softly caws. A faint amber light from outside, behind the shroud-heavy curtains.

Take more Ambien.

Up again. On the toilet. Nothing.

Move.

I realize, alone, it's happening again.

Shoulder-shaking Suzanna. Click on the light. 5:17. We have to go.

Off with the T-shirt. On with lecture clothes. Pants like lead. Shirt, an overcoat.

Water on face.

Suzanna beside me in the bathroom, flips on the light: "Are you sure?" she says.

I'm sure.

We hustle by the abandoned desk. The rental car starts, the first light is green, the next red, and I holler, "Just go! Just go!"

Suzanna speeds by the row houses, the narrow German-Amish lanes, predawn, looking for the H, spotting it under a yellow streetlamp.

"Just stop!" and I'm out, running for a door, any door.

"Excuse me. *Sir.* This isn't the entrance to the emergency room."

"Then where?" I say.

"What's wrong?"

"My heart."

"Your heart?"

"I'm sure."

"Do you need a chair?" Her Mexican face, her gold name tag.

"No, I can walk."

"Here, follow me."

She turns, strides. There's a beam emanating from her, her marching, the horse before the cart. Fall in step.

Coughing.

She turns. Starts to trot. "Come on!"

I trot, I come.

Clothes shed, electrodes stuck, five nurses swarming.

I hear, *his enzymes are elevated.*

I hear, *he's very hot.*

"It's a good thing you came in."

"I know," I respond.

"Been through this before, have you?" Another nurse asks—jocular tone, palliative irony.

"Yes—just not so far from home."

"Which is?"

I think Santa Fe. I say, "San Diego."

"You alone?"

"No. My partner dropped me off."

"A partner. Good. You've got someone to help you."

Greyhounds Chasing Rabbit • Again, the attending cardiologist tells me within ten minutes that I'm clogged, the right marginal artery (an offshoot of the right coronary artery) is blocked—again I need angioplasty—again I'm warned via angina and now this infarction, though it's milder than the first, says the interventionist, once (soon) he gets his probe up there, because, as he reminds me, the other three stents have kept their passageways open—again I would have died had I not been close to a hospital and someone brought me in—again there's damage (a heart attack *defined*) because the muscle's been blood-deprived—again, on the gurney waiting for the procedure or eating toast and drinking coffee the next morning, I feel this destinal salvation, right place/right time, luck and fate, crazy notions that nonetheless uphold a procedure the cardio team acknowledges was a "breeze"—and again I'm thrust back to the same/hardly-the-same existence for which, like a petri dish, my body has cultured another heart attack.

Before my cath-lab session on Saturday afternoon, after I've been stabilized on blood thinners, which is good news, since I'm not one hundred percent blocked. A male nurse asks if I would like him to pray for me.

My atheism is instinctual, so I say, "No thanks. I don't believe in that."

To which Suzanna pipes in, "You can pray with me." I see her willingness at once. Suzanna's praying, nothing like knee-dropping to God, but a faith in people and their collectivizing hope, doubtless has lightened the burden of her son's and grandson's illnesses *on her*: five years out and both of them are maintaining, mostly well.

I guess I should feel bad that I can't join their petitionary sorrow. But I don't. In that moment, I'm twitching with, let's just get the gurney moving.

I also wonder, during the eyes-wide, worry-long procedure, whether there's any other way to be with this condition, from now on, than my rooming in a Holiday Inn Express near a major urban hospital, my front-rowing myself at cardiology conventions, my donating blood samples and arterial cells and heart tissue, if possible, to the great cardio research centers of America (clinics Mayo and Cleveland), from which I'm offered helicopter service to the nearest cath lab, in short, some protectorate around my physical being so I'm never too far from the good doctors.

Batter Our Hearts • Post-op, I'm prescribed a spray bottle of nitroglycerin to replace the tablets, which, again, I nestle in my fanny pack like a derringer, holster-ready. The bottle is plastic, small, like nail polish, a red glass vial with a white top. Spray as needed under the tongue to assuage (you hope) the constrictive ache of angina—on your way to the E.R., of course.

Were there signs? Yes. The day of Obama's election I was visiting an old friend in Columbia, Missouri, where I first went to college in the late 1960s, and we went for a bike ride. I huffed and puffed, barely tackled the short rises, barely kept up with my buddy who circled back to check on me repeatedly. Out of shape, out of sorts, I toiled. Canceling that funk was the election-night exhilaration. No fatigue could pierce the ecstatic moment for me when W. was relieved of command.

Before we leave Lancaster on a preplanned trip to New York (the cardiologist says there's no reason I can't travel), the memoirists who brought me to Lancaster to lecture and teach take Suzanna and me to lunch. How relieved they are, I sense, that I didn't croak on stage. A framed photo of us seven arrives a couple months later. In it, I am puffy, a smiley face beneath two contrastively cast eyes—one, bewitched by the alacrity of the event, the other, jaunty and bright, as though nothing happened. My look is of two minds. I lean my right arm on the table; I want to feel fine (and I *do*) for the sake of these people and the trip, which continued. Next to me in the print, Suzanna has one untutored expression: *I wish I were anywhere but here.*

On to the city. From our perch on the Upper West Side, we treat ourselves to a play, a musical, the Natural History Museum, a backstage tour of the Metropolitan Opera, and a performance that night of John Adams's *Doctor Atomic*. I'm back in the saddle, in part, because we're moving. Suzanna motors on but complains, is fragile, wants to nap, get off her feet. Opera night, we eat at the Grand Tier restaurant. She consumes the spicy, expensive spinach.

In third tier seats, we hear a frenetic first act, the oxen pull of Robert Oppenheimer, the scientists, and the Army brass to build and detonate the atom bomb at Los Alamos. The highlight of the opening fifty minutes is Oppenheimer's aria, "Batter my heart, three-person'd God," from John Donne's *Holy Sonnets*:

> *Batter my heart, three person'd God; For you*
> *As yet but knock, breathe, knock, breathe, knock, breathe, shine,*
> *and seek to mend;*
> *That I may rise, and stand, o'erthrow me, and bend*
> *Your force, to break, blow, break, blow, break, blow, burn and*
> *make me new.*

Adams repeats "knock and breathe" twice as he does "break and blow." Augmenting the words seems to extend Oppenheimer's ache of conscience. His aria rises and descends on a chromatic pattern, suggesting, with its punctuated and slurred vowels, a staggering fall, a ravishing he longs for. I, too, feel ravished by the story, the score, and Adams's technique, still dazed by my Lancaster knockdown.

Just as the Act II curtain ascends, Suzanna taps my shoulder and says, "I need to get up. Walk around." What is it? Her stomach, she says. "I'll just stand back there," she points to where there's space. She sidles out. I espy her. She's pacing. Then gone. I get up and find her lying on a bench. All the benches, like the stairs and walls and seats and floors, are covered by the same luxurious red carpet, a sort of art bordello. She tells me to go back and sit down. She'll "endure" says her confused gaze. I sit, worry, turn to look. Her trouble is like mine, she's trying to will it away. I turn again. And then she appears: "We have to leave. Now!"

In a cab, up the tiny elevator, in the shoebox hotel room, and Suzanna is vomiting, a violent retching I've never heard from her. What is it? She doesn't know. Poisoned spinach? Later, I try to sleep, then hear the hurling sound and the toilet flushing. She doesn't ask for help. Honey, what can I do? Nothing, she says, and throws up again, the smell like a post-lunch grade-school boy's room.

By dawn, she's exhausted. Nothing left to purge. I've found a doctor online, an abdominal specialist on upper Fifth Avenue. We call, he'll see us, and we're off. At his office, his hands, massaging her stomach, tell him it's an appendicitis.

Seven hours creep by at Mt. Sinai Hospital (this, a week after my procedure, now hers just as serious as mine, the emergency bay she lies in a nuthouse, throated with hollering patients, some, we are told, wounded by gunfire), until, finally, the staff takes her to an operating room. It takes three hours for her laparoscopic removal, and he emerges, at last, with the news. "She had an abscess," he says, pushing up his sweat-wet, blue-paper cap, "very close to rupturing.

It took forever to get at it and not damage any other organ." He says he had to slice it into pieces then vacuum the remnants out. "The thing was gangrenous," he says. "It died a very slow death."

Next day I visit Suzanna in her private room and think how it's her time. To be sick. Then to be well. Her diseased organ has been surgically amputated; she's infection free, crisis tended to. Despite the takedown, I feel her trauma is passing.

In contrast, my recurring malady reveals an unexpected pattern. By which I mean a frame. While my condition's not acute, these past two-and-a-half years are bookended by infarctions, a palm-out *halt*—twice. That twice says my illness is chronic, albeit with a long/short passage in between its two ambushes.

Riding the six-square-foot elevator (the hotel's stent) to our floor and room, I'm alone, feeling pooled and boggy after a histrionic opera and an appendicitis. In the dark, seeking sleep, a vapory pall suffuses my body. Brooding burrows in. Each day, I find Suzanna woozy from her attack and eager to get out and do New York. I robot my way back to the hotel room, ponder each valve-off infarct. There they are, hiding behind the dunes, their scopes trained on my every move. *Christ, why now*, when my partner is not with me?

Twin Scares • Sunday, visiting hours are all day. Mt. Sinai's lobby is replete with a half-dozen elevators. I take the wrong one to the wrong eighth floor, stumble, retreat, then find the right wing and the right ride. I arrive at her room with the *New York Times* an hour before lunch. Happy to see me, she's still laid out, in bed and hospital smock. But, looking closer, I note a medicated lethargy in her eyes, espy a side table, wildly piled with stained pee bottle and ripped-open plastic packs and little orange vials, tops off.

She's uneasy; I'm uneasy. Neither of us can disguise it. No doubt, she's slept fitfully, jostling positions that intensify her incision's ache. I've been writing all morning in my journal about what's happening.

Suzanna sits up and grunts a bit. She refuses any I'm-in-pain moan. Still, she lifts her gown to show me the bandage over her three laparoscopic puncture wounds.

"Let's see yours," she says.

I unbuckle my pants. Beyond the gauze-covered catheter hole, the bruising radiates over my groin like an oil stain.

Our eyebrows arch weakly.

"What's in the paper?" she asks.

I cock my head at her, screw my eyes up.

"Susie," I say, grabbing a padded chair, "what's happening to us?"

"We're falling apart, are we not?"

"We are."

I'm worried that my father died following his *second*, five years after his first; my older brother, after his *second*, six weeks following his bypass—though Steve had to have had heart attacks prior to his big surgery. Why didn't I remember that their second infarcts disembarked as a matter of course?

"I've been going over this, this morning," I say. "I'm beginning to see that I should have been aware that this one was due—"

"Tom, that scares me." She reaches a hand toward me.

"And that I could have another."

I look at her hair smushed flat, that scoop neck part of the gown, skewed to one side and exposing bare, blotchy skin, her sudden frown. How worried she is for me. How worried I am for her. We've fallen into Alice's mirror in Wonderland. Being by *her* bedside turns it all topsy-turvy for me.

When I was in the hospital, the procedures and the doctor/nurse chats and the bloodlettings focused me, not on reflection, but on the healing at hand. A week later, with Suzanna the patient and me alone in a hotel room, I can't help but think about us, both ill, both aging, both moving toward death. All of which I don't want to lay on her—or think about myself.

"In Lancaster," I say, "after the heart attack and the doctor said we could travel to New York, I thought everything would be OK. And then after you got hit at the opera and the doctor said you'd be fine, I thought, again, everything would be OK."

"But—"

"But everything's not OK, is it?"

Hushed, I sense the stealthy breathing of death, its intimation of the nothing due, which will cool neither of us once it arrives. But right now she's healing because her appendix has been removed. Oh, would I have my problem, plumbed and removed! It's as if I'm the one in the hospital bed, though I've been coming and going on a cross-town bus, Westside/Eastside, another of the countless souls, searching for a bench in Central Park on which to waylay trouble.

I tell her I've been asking myself, what can I do? The strongest thing—taking her advice—is, Am I feeling it? That I've had a second *bad* heart attack? It seems it's *that*, which I have to feel, its throttling force, before I can get anywhere.

"I know that in my heart is where I'm supposed to feel this thing," I say, "but that's just it. When I go there, I find it's damaged, it feels less, and, besides, I can never know—"

"Never know what?"

"*When* the next one is coming."

Tears pool in the corners of her eyes. She smiles, embarrassed that the spigot just drips. I want to think Suzanna is crying less for herself and more for me.

She and I have merged. Look at her, see me. Until now, I never realized that the woman I love would receive and return so much of myself. That may be what I love about her. I used to think our separateness defined us. The road bricking up before us is the path of partnership, as wary as I am to admit the fact: one loads and carries the other's worry. My feelings embody hers. And she already has my worry pouring through her.

Stop! I can't keep us focused on so much dismay. Not now.

"Hey," I say, with faked zeal, "let me read to you what Maureen Dowd has to say about W's ouster."

Feelings I Know I Don't Know I Have • Home in San Diego, I hear from Dr. J's office that Lancaster Cardiology has sent my file. He wants me to come in. A quick hello, a handshake: pen tapping teeth, the balding Dr. J, my old and new charts refresh his memory. He reads aloud my total cholesterol number (150), ogles the stent photo (fine job), states my weight (205), schedules another stress test (Dobutamine echocardiogram), re-jiggers my drugs (back on Plavix so those platelets don't clump). He perks up to say that in Lancaster, *un-huh*, just one artery was stented, the blockage less than before at eighty percent.

It's odd, I know, but that figure hatches, for me, a benevolence—I'm progressing. The second clog is less. That twenty percent opening in my right marginal got me to emergency.

Un-huh.

To Dr. J I listen. I feel lumpy, belt-tight, befogged, as though my body has grown a sheath of fat to buttress the emotions this latest setback is demanding of me.

During a gap in his soliloquy, I note a framed photo on the wall.

"Who's that?"

"An old patient of mine, David George."

George, he tells me, bred thoroughbreds. In the picture, he's small, dwarfed by a horse and mounted jockey he's standing by, its neck wreathed with flowers at the Del Mar track. The horse won a high-stakes race that year, 1979.

"That was about the time he had his heart attack," Dr J notes. "He was fifty-nine. He knew it was coming, too; every man in his family had already died of the disease before sixty."

George's appointment in Samarra came promptly: a massive M.I. after which Scripps cardiologists stabilized him with Coumadin and without surgery.

"He's ninety now," Dr. J says, "still going strong." A rarity—a satisfied gleam in his eye.

"That's great. He knew the score."

"He knew."

I've learned that Dr. J—a photo of him, his hands on the chest of a heart-sick, bed-ridden man, graces the hospital lobby as part of a wall-mounted spread, celebrating the history of Scripps care—is a dedicated doc, numbers-driven, research-steady, the program-development type who's keen on treating congregations of heart patients, those pews of bad habits in the waiting room. Since he and his team rescued me, I regard him like a saint.

I state, "A pattern *I* should have known."

"Who can say," Dr. J offers, his register dropping to a well-deep doom. "The odds were not in George's favor. He certainly didn't have the benefits you have." In the moment, I smell the starch in his lab coat, the Purell on his hands. I sense I'm flat-out wrong. He's not a saint. He's my heart's judge. He's expecting something saintly of *me*—or my illness—which neither, so far, has given him.

He goes on: "Medications, stress tests, exercise, which you say you're doing, a vegetarian diet. So, yes, the odds were, you probably shouldn't have had another."

"And the takeaway is?"

"You did."

A look back at George's picture and wonder whether my face will grace Dr. J's wall one day.

In my car, I sit long enough to unpeel his last two words. *You did* wasn't said with judgment or prognostication. It was dismay. That was his tone. That's what I heard.

I start the engine.

I'm not there. Where I thought I was.

I'm repaired. Not fixed.

Feel it.

Feel how down, though not out, this condition has dragged me. And my body.

Feel how it has dragged me into my body.

Feel what it's asking me to do.

Feel this post-clog conversation Suzanna suggested I have with the me I *don't* know, this other, this *not* me, my body's me, my heart-hurt self, finally disclosing himself.

Feel how new this is.

How I'm Seen • We're at Harry's Coffee Shop in La Jolla, the big orange booth up front. My first time back, post-Lancaster. The faces of my men friends are warmly familiar. Bob, the oldest, who is rheumy-eyed like Andy Rooney; Mark, whose eyebrows rise involuntarily while he chomps his bacon; Marc, whose lips smack as he devours his oatmeal; and John, who eats the quickest, then pushes his ivy cap higher on his forehead, revealing age creases I don't recall.

The morning I'm back, they want my story. I tell them about the two lectures, four a.m. heartburn and chest pain, our run to emergency, one stent, one night in the hospital, our going on to New York, Suzanna's appendicitis at the Met, her operation—*and* we made it to *Spamalot*.

"Except for Suzanna," says Mark, "it sounds like what happened before."

"Yes and no," I say. "In retrospect it was much the same. But, of course, I didn't want to believe it could happen again."

I've ordered my usual: Swiss cheese omelet with tomatoes, no hash browns.

"Were there symptoms? Like before?"

I mention the bike-riding tiredness.

"Bingo," John says.

"What's the prognosis?"

"You mean, now that I'm twice reamed out? I wish I knew."

I see something then in their expressions: they mimic my unfazed attitude with their own—no surprise, no drama. Par for the course: Larson and his heart attack(s). Singular, plural, doesn't matter. If I don't quake with knotted nerves, they don't either.

I know John suffers from migraine headaches. During breakfast, he often shuts his eyes, puts thumb-and-fingers onto his forehead, and begins massaging, a signal that he's gone internal, where we don't tread. I've seen him clam up for a good five minutes and suffer like the proverbial war hero, in sick bay, waiting his turn. But then, while he checks out, we ramble on. Continuing the conversation is primary.

I say, "No, really, it was bad—that feeling of *Christ, not again*—and then it wasn't bad."

"What are the odds," Marc says, a statement, not a question.

"Well, they're different. There's having a second and there's dying from a second." I describe my father's and brother's short sticks. They surmised they'd cleared the hurdle after their first infarcts. As I did. Why wouldn't we?

"Since I didn't follow them to the grave," I say, "I beat those odds. But don't ask me about the odds for a third."

This line seems to hush them. I note a kind of frozen grief, as if to say each is calculating, agreeing that it's a very real possibility. *I'm a heart attack waiting to happen.* I recognize a glibness in my words, defiance, plus what I've noticed of late—how talking about my condition protects others who won't get close to the topic. I understand; it's theirs to avoid, not to commiserate with. Friends may regard this talk as contagious—as though the disease will rub off or their questioning me will set off "a third." Don't ask, and I won't tell.

They may think I'm the proverbial dead-man walking unless I ease their minds by saying I'm fine, I've got help, I'm working the odds and the drugs and the diet toward my favor. Yet aren't those the very things I did do after the first? I did, didn't I?

It's strange how there comes a time when *after the first* loses its mulligan. The next intersection is with what's coming. Not what I've survived.

Each of these men, I want to say, is dear to me, dear in that Friday-morning identicalness to last Friday, the laugh track of one's limericks, the expected nag of another's complaint about the high-priced menu, the shared disappointment we sometimes let fly about our children, the outrage we slip into for the wars of Bush/Cheney/Rumsfeld of which, if I gripe to Suzanna about their lynch-worthy crimes, she stops me cold, and says, "Take it up with the men!" and I do, the men corralling a kind of communal aggrandizement, so we're not just right in our persuasions but, even better, right among friends—I can't imagine being without my maleness, without the maleness of these men who accept my condition by not acknowledging the day coming when I'll be gone and they'll carry on the talking and forgive me my deceptions, my mulishness, for they recognize in *themselves* why I failed.

Mirrored in friendship, my heart attacks, as long as they are at bay, clarify more than they mire.

My Other Inner • One night I dream I'm in my office, at my laptop, trying to write this book, gut-and-head pain of some indeterminate nature nastier than normal, and I'm stopped for a long exhale, and I turn toward the mirrored closet door beside me and behind which I keep twenty boxes of personal files, my effects, notably my writing from the past three decades, and in the mirror I catch sight of another body in the room. I turn back to the screen. That other is me, proto Tom. Ripe, fit, whole, not fat. Eager, energized. Dressed in jeans, a rust-colored shirt, a jacket, sneakers, heading out, say, to do a reading of his new book or the multimedia lecture he's been writing to accompany it or the video essay he's begun dabbling in. "I'm all right," proto Tom says to me. His smile, so goddamned reassuring. I think/don't say: You're a lucky bastard. You'll survive me. You're living out the life *I* want to live out. May yet. Then, he's gone, my double. When I snap back, I don't remember if the pain went with the dream or with him, but my stomach is pond quiet. The dream returns, then, to its egg-laying bottom.

The Shape I'm In • It has taken a few years but about my disease I have, by now, written a lot. The memoirist's drawers bulge with new pages, as though my biography, whose ordinariness notwithstanding, is a full-plate venture for a future Robert Caro. But how do I begin to organize the pile? Start from the beginning. Which is where? My father's death? The genetic history he was given? The story of my infarction? How to tell the story of feeling great (loving my writer's life), feeling lousy, and the shifting degree by which my blood was/was not getting through?

Mulling such cause-consequent logic drives me bananas. Though I revisit the heart pain of my family, that hasn't in the least made me conscious of where I'm going. Only of where the

Larsons have been. If anything, grokking my past has made me . . . no, I can't justify that. I can't just manufacture a link between what I didn't know about the past with how much my not knowing has delivered the present.

One of my favorite southern California desert plants is the red barberry. It's a shrub that most years strains out a smattering of new branches, tolerates the sandy soil and brutal sun where it finds itself coming up year after year. Much of the plant's thicket dies in the desert's many rainless months. Its stalks grey and grow brittle. Winter sprinkles revive them. And by spring, its yellow flowers and red barberries begin festooning the clump. Unevenly. What I regard with excitable wonder every April is how the new blue-green leaves stipple the shrub in counterpoint to last year's dead parts. So the plant is what: Half-alive? Half-dead?

Looking at the red barberry, you're looking at how each species uses time to protect its space. You're looking at the interdependency of what has aged and died in the midst of what is reborn and reforming, of what has been against that which is new and never has been.

And the Barberry's Point • Were there a camera recording Tim Russert's death, no one would regard it aesthetically. It would seem, then, that dying has no artfulness—and yet how else do we view the top of JFK's head being sliced off by Oswald's bullet in the Zapruder film? He is scalped, right in front of Jackie who, horrified, crawls toward the secret service agents while the limo moves conspiratorially along. This brain-opening moment brought on a new category: a crossover from fiction to the unimagined, whose actuality (the film) needs no interpretation, whose millions of repetitions by viewers is its meaning. The tank-like unstoppable Caddie, the green hillock, the white pavement, JFK's blood on Jackie's pink suit. Beyond what a Nobel laureate could write. That rangeland where life and art lose their distinction.

Still, the moment of a heart attack is an amalgam of the artist's depiction and the patient's actuality. It's no wonder that my actual heart attacks seem cinematic, while acted out in these pages they seem real.

What it seems *is* what it is.

A memoir is a book you are writing about the life you have not quite lived.

One day, my few mourners, scattering my ashes on Santa Fe's Plaza, will say: Larson died as he lived, foundering in paradox. He may have been closer to wisdom than he knew. But why was the artfulness of his days not as apparent to him as it was to us, especially after he struggled to write this memoir? Maybe it was.

Theatrical • It's summer, in Santa Fe, a year and a half after Numero Dos. Suzanna and I are at the Lensic, a beautiful old refurbished movie house. We're watching the music documentary *Roy Orbison and Friends: A Black and White Night.* I learn later that Orbison died of a heart attack in 1988, age fifty-two, not long after this multi-rocker tribute was filmed. The stress of his comeback in the mid-1980s no doubt contributed to his sudden decline. There he is, singing "Oh, Pretty Woman," grinding out those interrupted guitar crescendos, satisfying his hopped-up audience with his lustful *growl*—when suddenly some Roy-like pulsing starts rising in my arms and chest.

I excuse myself, head for the bathroom. Always—to the bathroom.

In a corridor between two brick buildings, I feel very woozy, bloodless but standing. The walls aren't spinning but my lower body is shaky, weak-kneed. I think of my mother, how she feared *dying* in public. It's not the dying that troubles me, she said, it's the embarrassment. What an odd dread I thought, at the time, an old-world decorum that wouldn't let her just go but had to drag her, mortified, through propriety, one last Victorian bugbear of her generation. That mortified gawk in her eyes as she spoke, and I knew she was stone serious.

Holding to a railing, I run this movie through my mind. The actual final throes of my father and older brother haunt me. I fear falling to and writhing on the ground. Pounding my chest with clenched fist. Staring up at a circle of people and their tortured gaze, a man with a fedora and a woman with an umbrella, who whisper, "What's wrong with him?" to which I hope I'll shout back, "Nothing that your calling an ambulance wouldn't help." And one of the assembled, bending down, a Norman Cousins or good Samaritan, whose bigheartedness pushes him to say, "Don't worry, sir. You've got a strong heart. I can see it in your face. The ambulance is coming and all you need do is hang in there. Where are you from?" I tell him. "What do you do?" I tell him. "Why are you in Santa Fe? Oh, you used to live here and you love coming back. With whom? Your wife? Your partner. Where is she?"

And then, rising like Lazarus toward his aid, I want him to see inside me where what I dare not say pools like lava.

I don't want to die. I don't. I want to live. I want to live, and yes, knowing my death's been foretold. Please, listen. *Please*, spare me. Give me the chance to unbury what I've had to undergo these four years. I don't want to die now. *Christ, not now.* I don't want to go with so much unfinished. I don't want to abandon Suzanna to her son's illness and her own end. I don't want your ax held over my head, the firing squad, gunshot bulleting my skull—death, a great big Baby Huey who keeps saying *don't*-want, *don't*-want, *don't*-want, and I *don't* wanna be Zen about it and wager an OK, I accept whatever comes and promise I'll puddle uncomplainingly my splayed self on the pavement if, honey, you allow me one more chance to get the better of this before I get the worse.

How much this whining gums up my head, and, at last, I hasten to the bathroom—at least, to where I can close the stall door (no one would leave the film in the middle of "Only the Lonely") and make my peace *alone* with my dying or my faux death, whichever.

In the stall. Lock the door. Spray the nitro. Count to thirty. Feel the tremors lessen. *Are they lessening*? Yes, I think so. Try to unloosen my bowels. Nothing again and again nothing. Chew like a baby a baby aspirin.

I don't want to—not like *this*, frozen into submission, a George Segal sculpture, on a toilet seat.

And then like the air that vanishes under the parachute when the jumper tumbles on the ground, the billow subsides. The toll booth operator waves me through. I need no second spray.

I'm on my feet. *A first*: this—isn't—it.

When I sit down and smile/nod to Suzanna—she's unaware of what I've been through—I shake a bit. Not, I decide, with a heart symptom. But knowing full well that my imagination has terrorized me for seven minutes. It's intimidating, what I recently read—that one may "create" stress-induced angina: symptoms without the blockage.

How conspiratorial angina and its doppelganger are! The scenario I imagined I imagined away. There was no pain, only the tableaux. My brain—where my dying feels protected, downright sanctified, from my illness—ran with it, starting the prayers, enumerating the regrets, engaging all that man-overboard *this-is-it* malingering. Useless and necessary.

Orbison and k. d. lang sing "Crying," and I tell myself that yes, some constriction in my coronaries will flare up from time to time. And my brain (in part, my memoir-ness) stagecrafts a shadowy Act Five. Just a reminder. Of what's in store.

What Are the Odds? • By age sixty-five, one in ten Americans have had a heart attack. If a man has had one, the odds are *one in five* that he'll have another in six years; for a woman, it's one in three. The reason is, I'm finding out, coronary artery disease is not limited to one major heart-supplying blood vessel. Any of the three main coronaries can be clogged in one or several spots. The older you get, the more your chances of a second heart attack rise: from one in fifty-two, ages 45-54, to one in five, ages 85-94.

Of greater significance are the odds of dying with a second heart attack. They're much higher. Twice as many people die of a second or third attack than they do of the first. *Twice.* Of course, all these probabilities are worse if you smoke, eat crap food, ingest/make/retain pocks and pools of unstable plaques, don't medicate, don't exercise, don't lose weight, especially around the waist: big waist, small hips = unsound heart.

Although with my second attack my chances of escaping death were less, I nonetheless dodged the bullet. I find this curious. I was closer to death with the first heart attack, though my chance of having a first one was lower than my chance of having a second.

Am I spinning the prayer wheel? Does knowing the odds (versus not knowing them) change anything? Knowledge is supposed to free you so you make better decisions. But not-knowing, or being forgetful, is easy, natural, stress-avoidant. From it we are prone to marry early, buy lottery tickets, *not* hold 'em in Texas Hold'em.

And yet those odds of one in five aren't good. One in five is troubling.

What's more, all this is buoyed by my personality. One author friend tells me that, with illness, writers are less apt to *feel* our conditions since we over-dwell with the language-making energy of our minds. (I have, in the year after my second, written more than I ever have. A second book, a dozen new pieces. Since I think I'm closer to no longer being able to write, I do so rabidly.) We are also, my friend goes on, writing the ailment as it happens. Consequently, we are less *in* it than of it. There are times when this isn't so. Twice, on the way to emergency, doubling over in pain and fearing I'd die, my body was gunshot, collapsing on itself. But in between time, that is, the rest of my days, he's right: I'm "in my head" as a writer. Does this mean that if I get out of my head, I'll heal sooner? Is that possible? Would a non-analyzing, non-imaginative Thomas Larson still be me?

Am I just born with this strong head and weak heart? Is that my M.O.?

I don't know that the amount I think and write changes my health. Because it's my passion—writing my illness may help heal it. Because I experience more mental than emotional angst, my healing is negatively affected. Does that make sense?

When the condition is acute and present, I'm in it. When it's gone, I'm in my life. Which is not *it*. The trick, if possible, is to merge the two. But then a third rail arrives. The writer who shapes the separate spans of presence and absence differently. I write so that the heart attacks and their insight-rich aftermath are more meaningful than the time between them. Such occurs when I realize I can never comprehend my story. That's when the disease, my stand-in, my understudy, enters. He begins carving the story the persona of his disease insists he tell.

Three's a Charm • One Monday morning in April, I find myself in Scripps' emergency room, same place I was five years ago. My clothes are off, the gown's on, and I'm patched with adhesive pads and clipped-on cables for an ECG (also called an EKG). Results, negative. Next, bloodwork, or "labs." Only slightly elevated. Nothing too serious. They started a drip of Heparin, an anti-clotting drug, when I came in. I remain clammy and hot, close to basting. At home, 5 a.m. I was very hot, felt dopey and afraid, squirming with chest aches. I called the on-call cardiologist, Dr. H. He said come on in but don't drive, let someone else. Suzanna will, I said. Now, beside me, Dr. H is saying, *CSI*-like, "Tell me exactly what happened."

I awoke this morning vacant-headed and damp. I felt a tweaking rib-cage pain. I circle a trembling hand over my stomach. The drama of victimhood is always an aid. I sat on the john hoping a good crap would relieve me, but there was only the clamping-shut strain of a dead-force push. (Will I ever learn that my illness won't just *shit* itself away?) I lay back down in bed and felt some bestial alien opening its lizard eyes inside me. That got me moving. The kicker is—and Dr. H begins to nod—I woke up sweating at 5 a.m. A night's rest had not calmed the throbbing.

He says he wants to run an angiogram—shoot the dye up my femoral artery and see what my coronaries say. Something's constricted, he says, nodding with certainty. And we're off to the cath lab. I feel relieved, glad it was an actual symptom, glad I'm not a hypochondriac, glad I'm in the same hospital whose staff brought me back from the brink before.

In the bay, Suzanna is next to me. We await my turn, listen as a cardiologist two bays over speaks calmly yet forcefully to a woman he's preparing for angioplasty. Her voice is shaky, pleading; it must be her first. Please take away this pain in my chest *now*, not later, she says. He's whispering loudly, she, beseeching softly. I want to tell her how close she is to resurrection. But I think that a little fright is good for her. You'll be OK, he says; the symptoms will abate. Once we clean out your arteries you'll be surprised how much breath you'll have, how good you'll feel.

Like Walt Whitman, ministering in the hospital wards, Suzanna leans over and whispers in my ear, "Worst first."

A Russian nurse, Ileana, her face flat, blank, pretty, shows me a condom-like catheter. My member is shrunk but she smushes the rubber headpiece on anyway, managing to entangle pubic hair and scrotum flesh. When I examine it, the pubes pull painfully. I ask another nurse to fix it. She fumbles. I ask for a scissors. She doesn't have any. I tug and tug till it's free. Then I put a new condom on myself (for the next four hours not a drop of urine dribbles out). Ileana returns to shave my "groin area," telling me that soon they'll wash my "groin" before puncturing my "groin" with another catheter through which they'll insert the balloon and after which my "groin region" will be bruised and achy to the touch, so, she says breathlessly, don't touch it.

I lie in bed all morning, past lunch; Suzanna leafs the magazines. Three-thirty the call comes. A young Australian, shaped like a surfboard, wheels me through the swinging doors of the cath lab, the chilled inner sanctum of the hospital. We pass the cath "team" in their aqua blue scrubs, some with plastic shower caps indecorously skewed. They are relaxed but alert like a pit crew awaiting a NASCAR driver. They're my position players, specialists one and all, who introduce themselves: "Hi, I'm Jennifer, I'm Paul, I'm Ahmed." First they sterilize the "theater" where the angiogram takes place. Then they slide me from gurney to table top, a narrow altar on which for forty-five minutes three interventional cardiologists (one of whom is in training) wriggle that catheter into my "groin" artery, shoot in the contrast dye to measure the flow and pressure of my blood, monitor with picture and video the spidery mini-drama within, determine the amount and size of the blockage, say they'll ream it out, then insert a stent, what do you think? OK, I say, and then they push the balloon-catheter in, do the job, and cram in two stents, my inner roadways now with six total.

Again, with morphine and stents and blood flow, I feel serene. I land where I'm supposed to land. Having—No!—having *had* another heart attack. My third. A tripartite frame. My disease has, at last, included me in its call-to-arms. It's bighearted. It doesn't just bang open the swinging doors. It calls before coming. It's agreeable, considerate. *A Heart Attack Is Announced*, like some cozy Agatha Christie mystery. I hadn't thought of my condition as one which wants to harm me as much as it wants to give me a head start.

That night in my hospital bed, my crotch aches, I'm sated with water and juice, and the clock ticks, which, in its representation of time present, is soothing. In those beats (the romantic poet Novalis: "Every disease is a musical problem; its cure is a musical solution"), I hear the two directions I must take. Their paths are parallel, side-by-side. One is the path of unconsciousness, of sameness, of waiting for the next infarct, continuing what I've been continuing these five years and which has led to *this*.

I know that first path intimately. I was on it. I still am. I don't know the second. All I really have—how sweet to give in—is hope in what I don't know.

Remake the Past • In my hospital room, a physician's assistant, an officious, fleshy-faced woman, is reading off a list of reminders on my release form. It's the morning after my third angioplasty, and one night is all I needed. She's listing my six medications plus checking boxes: lower cholesterol, exercise, "watch your weight and your stress"—as in *reduce*.

"Stress," I guffaw. Knowing my third heart attack has been nipped in the bud and I'll soon be home, I'm glib: "I have no stress. I'm a writer. I wake up every morning and look forward to the desk—I love my work. It doesn't cause me stress."

Her quizzical look says, Are you done?

"Do you drive on the freeway?" she asks.

"Of course."

"Then you've got stress."

This, I later reflect, is said dismissively so we don't discuss it. It's also a warning: the lot of ordinary southern Californians, of which she's one as well, cannot escape their laptop prisons, their iPhone handcuffs. Sedentariness only worsens a heart condition. Stress is ubiquitous.

I want to repeat all this for Suzanna when she picks me up. But instead, getting me in the car, she can't wipe away her ghastly look. She says, "Do you know the interventionist sought me out last night before I went home? He wanted to tell me that the artery he opened was the widowmaker. Your attack could have been 'fatal,' he said. He was shaken. I could tell. There was a heaviness in his voice. I was stunned. Just like the first time."

The widowmaker. The Tim Russert artery. Mine was not *fully* blocked as his was. Another great escape.

That afternoon, Suzanna and I are sitting in our sunroom, the tall-windowed addition to our house. We're exhausted, and the unobstructed view across the pool and the canyon and the trees on the opposite mesa a quarter mile away is calming.

We sit close, separate chairs but angled toward each other.

"You know what I've been thinking about?" I say, sitting back. "My mother. A year or so before she died, she called me one day to say she was 'walking up a short incline' in Atlanta and felt a stabbing pain. It was, her doctor said, angina. I said, 'Angina? Wasn't that Dad's thing?'

"A week later I flew in and drove her to a Cincinnati hospital for her angioplasty. I remember her deference to the doctor—he looked a lot like Dr. J—our doing a crossword puzzle together while a nurse stanched the bleeding in her groin where the balloon catheter went in. Her cardiologist told me he unclogged the block, taking it from eighty percent down to zero."

(All this I had just read, a few weeks before, in my 1991 journal.)

"How childlike she was," I continue. "Her eyes pleading with me, her voice drifting into a kind of girlish singsong, 'Please, Tommie, I left my thinking cap at home; you need to help me find the words,' in the crossword."

That single moment rattles and dizzies me. I enfold my hands, put them to my mouth, close my eyes. Suzanna puts her hand on my knee.

"I don't know how my mother lived with the deaths of Steve and Dad. And then to have it compounded by her own scare?"

I remind Suzanna that despite my mother's successful surgery, it allowed her depression to come to the fore. She seldom named her fears. But she did broadcast her symptoms. She would say, "Tommie, I don't have any pep. Not like I used to." That's how I knew something was wrong. My sense is, she spiraled into a kind of genetic nihilism. *Laden with so many problems, there's nothing I can do.*

Oh, the questions I was unmindful to ask her. Did she think how Dad's condition, and then hers, may have doubled their sons' risk of cardiovascular disease? (How much of this will show up in my boys, now men?) Did she realize only after her anginal episode that she, too, might suffer a heart attack? Was she not drawn to analyze the disease's origin—because, within two years, another invader began menacing her chest. After forty years of smoking, she was diagnosed with lung cancer, a death sentence that outpaced any narrowing of her arteries. Six months later, she was gone.

"She had some form of heart disease," I say. "Our parents passed us a double dose."

"Another pattern at work?" Suzanna asks.

"For me, it's something else. The doom I felt—we all felt—that our family—everyone—was cursed." As she and I lace our fingers together, I sense something is becoming unstuck.

And yet that pile of cholesterol *didn't* appear out of nowhere. "The fat my father and my brother and I carried," I say, "we ingested." I describe our move to Wisconsin in 1959 where the pounds piled up: A&W-root-beer-float-ham-sandwiches-Dairy-Queen-banana-split-buttered-mashed-potatoes mounded our plates, at home, at school, at restaurants, at Grandma's house. We swallowed tablespoonfuls until every blood passage in our lazy-bones bodies was bumpered with hardening heaps of plaque.

"Honey," I say, "I'm still overweight. This *goddamn* fat is still plaguing me." I feel a sudden sorrow for that adolescent boy who, to escape his family and his fate, hoped to tie his arms and legs to the bed and stretch away his legacy. As though *he* were a fetus I keep trying to abort.

"And I'm right," I say, "that this was my parents' genes coming out in their sons' bodies."

The realization that I knew this all along and the moment that says I am just now barreling through the saloon doors swings open.

"This is the pattern," I push on. "Every time I have one of these attacks, I've got to reconfigure my past."

"Do you think that's what's being asked of you? To remake your past?"

"In part, yes. In part."

We both ease back in our chairs.

All this—one day after heart attack number three—the widow-maker, but only partially blocked.

In part elbowing *partially*.

Which is also elbowing *partnership*. We. When Suzanna and I are close, I'm safe, secure. Safe and secure in her touch, her companionship, her simply being with me, with my questions, my memories. Simply being.

Her blood fills my heart. We are much more than each other's mirror.

Plus, my six-stented ticker—not like a teenager's but, nonetheless, buoyant again.

In lieu of an altered fate, the gift of change, wrapped and ribboned.

And isn't *this*—partnering on with Suzanna—what I want to live for?

FOUR

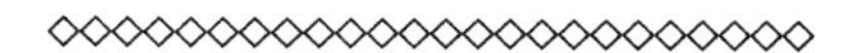

Why did all this wisdom and beauty have to come so late?

— Anatole Broyard, "Journal Notes,"

Intoxicated By My Illness

What More Can Be Done • A week after the interventionist scaffolded my arteries with a fifth and a sixth stent, Dr. J and I are again in one of the little cubicles of Scripps cardiology. I'm on the short bed with the black-leather covering. With my file open in his hands, he is saying, like a mechanic coming out from underneath the hood of a car, that because I'm on the requisite drugs—aspirin, a statin drug, and five others: I tell friends I'm a ward of Pfizer—and that because the pharmaceuticals are doing what they're supposed to—blood-thinning, heart-rate-slowing, anti-blood-clotting, bad-cholesterol-inhibiting, good-cholesterol-raising, blood-pressure-controlling, inflammation-lowering—and that because six stents are positioned in the proximal, or sturdiest, segments of my coronary arteries, "We've done all we can for you."

What?

He means, if I catch his drift, they fixed the problem I brought them to fix: an exploded plaque. That's what they do, the interventionalists, his pronominal *we* indicating a collective task.

His remark is a jolt. Here you go, the tire's plugged, the tank is gassed. Keep going. Travel on. Where am I going, though, with a patched tire and a dropping fuel gauge? I thought *where* was into the treasure chest of the rest of my days, gems and doubloons still heaped. I thought angioplasty and stenting would extend my time. But this is a fool's errand. (In ninety percent of stented heart patients, the hardware does nothing to stop another attack. Any retooling erodes over time. Scar tissue forms at the site of the stents as well as at the site where heart-muscle cells died during an infarct.) All I am is extended for however long the repair lasts. Despite the new treads, the Toyota has 200,000 miles on it. With each angioplasty, my expectation is revived and diminished; I'm worn down and resilient. This slippage back into the "conundrum of heart disease"—well, OK, but *Christ*, I'm tired of it. How many times must I bell-ring the paradox: my arteries are on the verge of clogging shut, but without symptoms of said shutting, nothing's imminent.

I thought I'd have a sell-by date, meaning an *end* to my heart disease would arrive. I'd be fully disenthralled. Such is the ease of the ego, my inner James Gandolfini.

If anything, my disease has been renewed, as though it's a library book I get to keep a bit longer.

Perhaps the definition of an illness is that after you hear your doctor say he's done all he can, the disease is truly, finally, existentially yours.

A Dreaming Lipidologist • A month goes by following my third post-infarction checkup with Dr. J. It's spring, and Suzanna and I have escaped California again for New Mexico. In Santa Fe, at a laundromat, I find a poster announcing a series of talks by a "board-certified lipidologist": "Artery Disease: Beyond the Cholesterol Number." The description says that advanced lab tests and ultrasound studies are "tragically underused" in the treatment of this disease. Suddenly, I think I've found someone whose alternative practice may complement Dr. J's, who has, I remind myself, done all he can do.

At a community center, I hear Dr. M talk. He's a Ponderosa pine of a man, walrus mustache, cowboy hat on the table, approachable, holistic. Like many newcomers to Santa Fe, he's thrilled to be here, after his mutually-agreed ouster from a fourteen-floor HMO in Philadelphia. His summaries of statin drugs and their side effects, plus new links between Alzheimer's and heart conditions, are tantalizing. We make an appointment.

In his office (there's no assistant, just him and two small dogs), I ask if I can use a tape recorder. No problem. He has me describe my plight and the experts involved. He characterizes my Scripps man, Dr. J, as a "big study and consensus cardiologist," who is "reactive rather than preventive." When the field is so dominated by those HMO guys, it's one reason why, as a cardio-activist, Dr. M has opened a cholesterol studies and treatment practice in Santa Fe—to treat the person, he hopes, before the infarction.

He says yes, opening his oak desk drawer for a plastic-wrapped blood-draw hypodermic needle, that there's always something new to uncover about the nature and extent of one's disease. He recommends a blood test to measure cholesterol particles (there are nine sizes), and target the worst LDL with supplements.

First, tests.

Dr. M scans the carotid artery in my neck. He finds no new plaques and a few old ones. He says this gauge has a ninety-six percent correlation to the coronary arteries, meaning neither my carotids nor my coronaries have new plaques. He measures my IMT or intima-medial thickness. The intima is the entire arterial wall, including the endothelia, the most intimate part of the intima, against which the blood moves. One doctor has described it as "a single pavement layer of cells." (Endothelia cells are remarkable multitaskers. They make a gas called nitric oxide that widens the passageway, inhibits most cholesterol from sticking, and holds down inflammation. In the coronary arteries that surround the heart, the endothelia surface is silky smooth. [Its width is in nanometers, thirty to seventy billionths of a meter.] Blood barrels through. However, after years of one-way traffic, the endothelia cells show the wear and tear. The worst is when small bits of cholesterol penetrate the arteries' lining and collect into plaques.) My thickness is .71 mm, optimal for my age. He does a blood-pressure dilation test, placing the cuff around my arm and leaving it pumped up for five minutes. This forces the artery to dilate in my forearm, which he scopes with the ultrasound wand. The artery opens to sixteen percent: above five percent means I have, statistically, a zero percent chance of having a heart attack in the next five years.

None of these things did Dr. J do or suggest.

"Seems like I'm in good shape."

"Those stents may have done the trick," Dr. M says.

Over several visits, I come to admire Dr. M tremendously. His desk-side manner. His genuineness. His touch. He ultrasounds the arterial pressure in my ankles, my feet resting on his blue-jeaned leg. He applies too much goop, then wipes the excess on his jeans. One dog, cuddled on his bean bed, sighs and shudders back to sleep. Dr. M typically spends sixty minutes with me, perhaps since I like "discussing lipids."

One visit, he tells me a story about a friend, another lipidologist, who stole the show at a recent cardiologists' convention by talking not about statistical assays among control groups but *personally* about the case histories of her diseased patients, men and women who changed her as much as she them. Before finishing the tale, he choke-pauses and says, "Right now, I've got a big lump in my throat just thinking about it." And, on preventive vs. reactive medicine, he says: "A lipidologist is one who dreams this stuff. You wake up at three in the morning, thinking that article has overlap with that patient you saw last week, then you write stuff down at the side of the bed. The cardiologist, on the other hand, is *woken up* at three a.m. because someone's at the hospital who's just had a heart attack. The point is, there's space for both."

I love his inclusiveness. Such a new thought, too. The fact that I don't have to decide among treatments.

He takes my blood and says he'll send it off for a range of cholesterol tests.

Later, as I listen to the tape, I hear Dr. M state that we all need to "think more about cholesterol." Countering heart disease lies in increasing the body's efficiency, "to enhance cholesterol delivery to, and removal from, the cells," he says. How can we help "the cholesterol-logged cell" advise "the body to get rid of it? What's best? Drugs? Plants? Exercise? Fish oil? All those?"

In my files, I locate copies of blood-test notes by Dr. G, my physician during the 1990s. In 1996 and 2000, he writes, "Your cholesterol is higher." Those times, my totals were 246 and 261: dangerously high. "This," Dr. G continues, "indicates more fat and sugar in your diet. Please decrease both. Consume more fish and white meat and less beef, pork, and lamb. Eat fruits, vegetables, and nuts such as almonds and walnuts. Eat olive oil instead of butter and margarine. Exercise at least 40 minutes every day." Good advice. Except I'd been a vegetarian since 1984, albeit a dairy-loving, sugar-and-starch one. All through my forties and fifties, I gained weight, ran up sky-high cholesterol numbers, and did nothing about it.

This is proof that fat sticks to and punctures my coronary lining more so than most people. It doesn't matter that my second and third clogs and infarctions were less severe than the first attack. Any amount of plaque draws added fat to it like flypaper. Maybe if I consume no fat, I'll not be fat.

The message adds up. Heart health is not achieved with stents and pharmaceuticals alone. They are crucial. But cholesterol is the real enemy. *My enemy.* I listen. Tests. Exercise. Diet. Supplements. Just as I'm buoyed by Dr. M's explanations, I also hear him suggesting I change. Although I'm not used to taking charge—I'm used to being fixed—it feels as though three interventions have changed me.

Suddenly I parachute into a clearing where my disease and my health are conferring and asking me to referee.

No-Oil Vegan • The one practical thing left *to* do? Change my diet.

As I've said, I've eaten so much *cow* that my insides are plastered with casein, a milk protein adult humans digest poorly. It's as though casein's mutagenic coagulants bedevil my stomach, a witches' cauldron of insoluble fat, sticking to my arterial lining. I thought I'd cut down/cut out all that poison. But it snuck back in, in the everything's-made-with cheese, eggs, milk. Long ago, quitting my two-pack-a-day cigarette habit, my lungs eventually ousted the nicotine killer. But it took years. Vegetarianism, while good for the planet, made me fat and unhealthy.

Suzanna finds Dr. Caldwell Esselstyn's *Prevent and Reverse Heart Disease* (he describes heart disease as "food-borne illness") and T. Colin Campbell's *The China Study*. The film, *Forks Over Knives*, debuts. We read. We watch. We scour labels. They say the same thing. No animal protein. No nuts. No fats of any kind. A plant-based diet, they insist, adds negligible cholesterol.

I decide: I'm vegan. Soy milk. Legumes. Fruit. Vegetables. Whole grains. Nothing else. Plus, according to Esselstyn, I need to do without the one ubiquitous ingredient that all heart patients should avoid (and I've never avoided)—oil. A no-oil vegan.

This last shift is the hardest. Who knew that in America almost all processed and cooked foods, whether made fresh or packaged or lying in tubs in the deli, has oil. It takes twice as long as before to label-hunt our way through Whole Foods and Trader Joe's: and there, on the most divinely innocent foods, like Gluten-Free Vegan Soy Burgers, is safflower oil or canola oil or extra virgin olive oil. Put it back. Can't have.

Except for a few things like sourdough bread, Ezekiel cereal, coffee, chai, strawberry preserves, vanilla soy milk, everything else is raw.

One night, Suzanna, who is mostly on the vegan diet with me, says to the ice-cream server at a dinner party and pointing at me, "I don't eat dairy because of him."

No indigestion, no duplicitous heartburn/angina, no bloating. Now, was that so hard?

Stress Echo • Later that summer, we're back in San Diego. There, at the hospital, shirt off, chest swabbed, electrodes attached, I lie down for my annual checkup, an echocardiogram, a two-stage procedure. First, the echo technologist goops a wand with gel and rolls it across my chest, my heart at rest. She takes four ultrasound videos, close-ups of the four chambers. Next, I walk for twelve minutes, faster and faster, on an incline-raising treadmill. My heart pumps madly, I stride and push, grasp the bar, a sailboat rail in rough seas. I lie down, and she ultrasounds the organ again. (I've pushed my resting rate from 69 beats per minute to an agitated 151.) The moving images record what's termed "wall-motion abnormality," that is, my heart-attack-weakened muscle cannot respond with full vigor as it once did.

Post-stress, on my back, I spot on the screen the damage from my initial heart attack five-plus years before. Its grizzled grey mass is eerily spectral like moonlit fog. I ask, "Can that be repaired?"

"You'll have to speak to the doctor about that," says the tech.

I think, well, of course; techies can't diagnose, at risk of lawsuit; so she defers. Schooled woman. System-protective system. But I want answers. Or reassurance.

"Your heart," she does offer, perhaps seeing my muzzy look, "is contracting and expanding well." In the image, she says, she's searching for "wall thickening" in the left ventricle. Thickening means the heart muscle inflates with sufficient blood to squeeze and send blood—the ejection fraction—into the arteries. A robust ejection is what you want.

The attending cardiologist, a Chinese woman, enters. She reads the screen before sending the pictures to Dr. J, who will interpret them with me/for me later. Still, I ask, "Can that gray patch be repaired?"

"No," she says.

Ah, the truth.

"But," she hastens, "there's nothing here to worry about."

Huh? If part of my heart's dead, how is there nothing to worry about? My heart, relaxed, starts pounding again. I squirm on the paper I'm lying on, paper like a Denny's place setting. I strain my neck to see into the image but I also regard the Chinese doctor, her perfectly clipped raven hair, a tiny silver cross dangling against her alpaca sweater. What do I want from her? She's told the truth. Why do I think she or other health care professionals owe me anything more?

When a copy of my echo report arrives, I spend a morning underlining all the pertinent phrases, Googling them for definitions, trying to grok its jargon. An hour of holding my head up on the desk as if it were a bowling ball on a table, and I write it out in my journal.

Some of the phrases seem alarmist to me. "Abnormal resting electrocardiogram"; "abnormal stress echocardiogram"; "no new stress-induced wall motion abnormalities"; "flattened inferior-lateral T waves at baseline with non-diagnostic inferior Q waves"; LV (left ventricle) wall motion at rest "mid-apical lateral wall hypokinesis" and "mid-basal inferior wall akinesis"; LV wall motion under stress "mildly hypokinetic" and "inferior wall remains akinetic from mid to base"; "global systolic function is mildly reduced."

Damage to my heart muscle after three heart attacks is, I estimate, ten to fifteen percent. A chunk of my left ventricle, the harder working of the two, has decreased mobility; it's hypokinetic. That chunk is motionless; it's akinetic. That's why, when I walk up four flights of stairs or hike at 8,000 feet, I'm breathless.

The truth rears: Nothing's changed in five years. Although, I am alive.

I want to tell Suzanna I'm barely treading water but I don't. I retreat, saying, "You know, I've got a shitload of online papers to read." I spend the weekend in my office, map the results of my echo with red, green, blue, and black pens. Though I'm blue-black woozy figuring this stuff out—I do it anyway. I cup my face and stare at the diagram, no more penetrable than if I stared at my chest, trying to see my coronary plaques.

One week, then another, creeps by. I'm back in the cardiology waiting room, my foot-shaking a nervous pulse on the carpeted floor. I keep rereading my notes, my colored grid.

It's then I finally hear the all-caps phrase at the report's end shouting at me, an emergency siren pushing through this diagnostic snowstorm: CHRONIC ISCHEMIC HEART DISEASE.

My disease is *chronic*. It's here to stay—and it's going to kill me. It's here *to* kill me. Perhaps not tomorrow. But sooner not later. That's what the no-comment techie and the nothing-to-worry-about doc were saying. By not saying it.

Ushered into the cubicle, I wait twenty minutes for Dr. J. He enters briskly, shakes hands, and I'm thrusting him my data—diagrammed, red-underlined. Soon I shut up, defer to him, as always. When he talks—the illness is more salient than the patient—I hear that my arteries are as wide as they can go, the large, ruddy sump of my heart that's working is working well, there's no sign here of an impending wreck. I think of this loquacious man, often overwrapped in his intellect, who is also making compassionate little speeches to frightened heart patients every day.

Then something happens, the thing I don't know. Dr. J ear-plugs his stethoscope to listen to my heart, and his talking stops. One hand palms my shoulder, the other guides the floating silver disc on my back and chest. The long quiet is basementy, conspiratorial. His concentration, submarine commanderly. I sense we're breathing as one, Lamaze-like. Then, his admission—"the sound of that thump is quite strong"—and I feel cared for, immensely cared for.

Push the numbers back. Bury my penchant for them.

What am I feeling? *What your condition is asking you to do.*

My heart—its blast-scar irreversible—wants consoling. Wants to be attended to. Wants to be seen, wants to be heard. Much as it was that frightful first night I rushed in: *I need help. I'm having trouble breathing*. How elastic that need I had to be attended to stretches then to now. To be consoled, comforted, assured, listened to, more than talked at. Commiseration to match the infarct anvil I'm carrying.

My thump felt, it is, for the moment, as it was before. (Not as it ever shall be.) The heart—for a long moment—recalls its adolescence, its strength and verve, its cocky attitude, its full-bloodedness—a first baseball glove, parents leaving me at college. This turn back spites the ever-narrowing passageway.

I also realize I need to participate more with what I want to happen than what I fear will. I'm called in. I'm medicated. I'm treated. I'm done. Lifesaving yes, but it's not good enough. Let the numbers go. Let intimacy, as rare as it is, ravish me. Love it for its one-night stand, its lottery-like unlikelihood. Let it linger as long as it can. Be thankful it's not any less. Be the person being seen, being heard, hope outweighing diagnosis.

So, for the rest of our session—the thirteen minutes HealthNet stipulates we get twice yearly—I'm clutching our give-and-take like a piglet on the teat. *The sound of that thump*. I seem to float up to the ceiling and observe us.

From there, I'm performing a bit, though not falsely. I want him to notice my softening. I want my passions to stimulate his. His, mine. I listen, put my notes aside, ask whether there's any procedure yet invented for any cardiologist to detect an unstable plaque in the arteries? It's like feeding a sardine to a seal.

"You mean," he replies, "if we could send a catheter up there and see the plaque that's going to burst next Saturday at two in the afternoon? If I knew how to do that, I'd get the Nobel prize in medicine." A ticklish laugh sidles out.

I'm nodding at Dr. J like a groom to the preacher. Surely, he knows what patients want. *The surfacing, the buoyancy, lingering above water, not dying, saved.* I feel I must care about him as well. Such things he can't give he knows he can't, and I accept that.

Outside the hospital, I fall to my ritual gloat. I get coffee, now with soy milk, sit and admire the fact that my next blood test is three months off. I'm content. Exiting the parking lot, I recall a statistic I forgot to mention: of the ninety-two percent (back to numbers) of heart patients who have angioplasty, take medications, eat good food, and work out—ninety-two percent do *not* have a heart attack in the five years after their *first.*

Their first. But I had a second. I had a third. This stat doesn't represent me. No, it *does*: I'm in the eight percent. Such numbers are like relatives staying on, uninvited.

That's when I'm hit by one of Dr. J's pronouncements: *Your arteries are as wide as they can go.* TL's in the eight percent, and he's at the widest width possible. Isn't this what he told me last time, before I went to Dr. M—*We've done all we can for you*?

Christ, I didn't ask what he meant, so busy was I under a spell. Are my arteries as wide as they are because my left ventricle pumps only so much? Is it because the ventricle is forcing its eighty-five/ninety percent capacity to flex harder than before? Is it because arteries can't repair themselves and are fated, post-heart-attack, to compress like a python digesting its prey?

To what degree am I fixed? Unfixed? Unfixable?

The tizzy rises. Hands palm the steering wheel. Numbers nag me nutty. If I want an answer to this indeterminateness, I won't get it desiring the determinable.

The only thing I can count on is his touch, Suzanna's, Dr. M's, awakening me. That if I widen my heart's yearning to connect, I—along with the vegan diet, the cleansing pills, the yellow-highlighted stats—will steady those wall-motion abnormalities, relax that coronary constriction. There's so much and so little the medical people can do. The rest is mine. My health is mine. My disease is mine.

In "The Patient Examines the Doctor," Anatole Broyard writes, "I just wish he [the doctor] would *brood* on my situation for perhaps five minutes, that he would give me his whole mind just once, be *bonded* with me for a brief space, survey my soul as well as my flesh, to get at my illness, for each man is ill in his own way."

I doubt Dr. J realized it but he did *get* at my illness, if only briefly. The other half is, I took his *getting at* and made it about me. Our bonding space was stethoscopic, our "five minutes" closer to one. That halcyon familiar. *My heart being heard.* The moment I felt his heart go out to mine. Indeed. Physicians survey souls. They can. Too bad they seldom do, though I'm saying now that this, in addition to the intervention, is what we patients and our wandering souls want.

Thoughts That Just Occur • The immediacy of an actual heart attack cancels time. One week of stress brings it on, its reckoning barges in, you're treated via miraculous interventions, and you survive. Another heart attack follows, and another, and voilá, there's a pattern. The repeatability and the smooth contour of that pattern makes the time in between—blown away, built back—feel destinal. In rumination, time bends, and there, fear-flagged thoughts rush the stage in droves.

That the distance I am from a full-service hospital is long (an hour, say)—I'm visiting friends at the top of Michigan's lower peninsula or driving across southern New Mexico—and there's no recourse except to indulge this thought and try (and fail) to dismiss it.

That when I awake at four a.m. from a robust dream with what feels like a tightening chest, it may be only the dream's fear manifesting itself in my body, an imagined angina in my ghost heart.

That a heart attack sets onc adrift, similar to how Roger Rosenblatt describes the uncharted tack of grief—moving "in the direction you least trust."

That when I tell people I've had three heart attacks—I mention my disease at a weeklong writing seminar in Bethesda, Maryland, and a woman says, "Is there something about you we should know?"—the pained, thwarted look of friends, colleagues, students, and strangers means they don't know whether to caretake me, resent my admission, or let it go.

That the future and the past blend in this nonterminating present.

That one of my favorite poems, Donald Hall's "White Apples"—which begins, *When my father had been dead a week / I woke / with his voice in my ear*—echoes just after an infarct, my father beckoning me to join him in the nest of crocodiles. The damaged heart, a white apple.

That over the five years my disease has skirmished with me, I've had just a few honk-eliciting stalls and the rest of the time the van has motored cleanly through the tunnel.

That I know no other way to miss the time coming when I'm not alive and Suzanna is alone than by feeling *her* fearing its arrival while I'm still here.

That head pain (anxiety, malingering) accounts for fifty percent of emergency room visits for chest discomfort and breathing difficulties, i.e., infarct false alarms, nonetheless terrifying.

That walking the ledge of the Grand Canyon's North Rim, 8500 feet, one day, dropped me dizzily to my knees, breath-catching on bellowed lungs, transmogrifying the airless realm—same thing shook me long ago in Machu Picchu, under its bell-jar sky—insisting to Suzanna that I was expiring like the little fish flipping over and over on the dock, gasping for its element in Ross McElwee's film, *Time Indefinite.*

That terror is rare while the past remains worrisome and relieving.

That Tim Russert's plaque crack took him from a symptomless fifty percent occlusion to a head-on collision, and *swoosh*—it's time to update the Wikipedia page.

That I'd rather be sick and with Suzanna than be without her and not have the illness.

That I'd rather have no book than lose her.

That to be entangled in not wanting the book to end is to be nearing its completion.

That the plaque-clearing interventionist cardiologists achieve apes the mind's clarity when the plaque of self-deception is Moses-parted with stents of ambiguity, uncertainty, humility.

That in college I loved reading Lionel Trilling, the august left-wing New York intellectual, who links literature and society with a moral passion like no other critic, and who, after he finishes reading a novel, peppers himself with the ethical question, "What does this book want me to do?" What does my heart disease want me to do?

That I was ill and now I'm not is incorrect: I've *always* been ill.

That not dying conjures up Whitman in *Song of Myself*: "All goes onward and outward / nothing collapses, / And to die is different from what any one supposed, and luckier."

That not being sick, how swiftly inured I am to not being sick.

That my twin sons, now in their thirties, know of my attacks but don't/can't know what they're in for.

That I wish I could have involved them more in my disease and in my recovery. Around them, I hated being a malingerer, seldom said how troubled I was. I wanted to be the change, dwell on neither the ups nor the downs I endured. I realize now, that was unwise. I wish I had spoken up (perhaps this book is my *speaking up*), been thornier, unruly, ailing. So they could experience the inflamed me. But who wants to be the sickly one? In their thirties, my sons are fit, with low cholesterol, mostly vegetarian, free of the symptoms of heart disease. So, too, was I at their age. They could get a cardiogram, but doctors shy away from ordering one unless you're symptomatic; my sons' cost would be out of pocket. They could take a statin drug if a doctor felt it necessary. For their birthday, I promise to buy each an analysis of their genetic history, their "disease ancestry" from "23andMe." (It's a self-administered DNA test, done via mail.) Will a warning of inevitable coronary artery disease incite their awareness? I like to think such knowledge would have made me an advocate. But too often I was wrapped up in my quotidian life to be aware of my health.

That death is not the end of endlessness, for there is no I-will-be-here to realize that my endlessness is over.

And, finally, that we recalcitrant ill are like Janet Leigh in *Psycho*—fleeing Phoenix with embezzled cash to roll on the bed with her shirt-off lover, the rain pounding the windshield, the wipers flapping at the sheets, a flashing MOTEL sign pulling her over, hauling her in as victim. Which Leigh never sees coming. Why should she? She's an outlaw; her blindness is her character. Which she also can't see, for she keeps glancing into the rearview mirror. When a heart attack drags you down the stairs and out on the lawn, screaming for help, there's a score playing, much like Bernard Herrmann's music. But we don't hear it. It's just too terrifying to be aware of the prelude's feverish urgency, announcing the knife thrusts coming in our own lives.

Running from the Family • Six years younger, my brother Jeff remembers Dad and Steve and their heart disease not as familial myth where I elevated them, but as out of control and abusive. He's a scientist, a water biologist, who also reads and writes Civil War historical novels. He calls one day to tell me he went to the doctor a few months ago. He was terrified that he couldn't stop eating Mickey D's and drinking diet cokes. He was up to six sodas a day. He knew he was condemned to sluggishness by the Larson gene. He got on the scale, and lo, there it was: 252 pounds! He quickly calculated his BMI: he was *obese*. A word with the lexical criminality of other epithets shouted by bullies from passing cars: Shamu! Lardo! Five-by-Five! It's appalling to admit, but my dad, a porker himself, called our homegrown fuck-up of an older brother, Steve, who scaled in at 280 in high school, "Buckets." *Buckets.* And now Jeff's obese, the most motivating and despair-ridden word in all of Fatland. But wait. Though he's been doomed to the club, he's out. He has, he says breathlessly, adopted plant-based meals and lost forty pounds! Forty pounds? Forty pounds. In three months. (Three months later he will have lost fifty-seven pounds!) You're kidding. He's not. Just plants? Yes, plants, mostly. I can't believe it. But I should. I've been on the same regimen, eight months now. I've been losing weight as well. I'm getting it, particularly what T. Colin Campbell means when he writes, "Nutrition controls the expression of genes." The nutritional healing a plant-based diet activates is the missing link.

Off the phone, I convey the good news to Suzanna, wonder whether my journey has anything to do with Jeff's weight loss, and she says it does—he wised up because of my heart attacks. How old is he? she asks. Fifty-seven. One year older, she says, than you and your father were when you had your first ones. (Suzanna's relational laser tracks such things.)

"He's awake," she says.

"I really motivated him?" I say. "I don't believe it." I explain that if so it means he did something no Larson has ever done—listened to the family's heritage.

"That may be important," Suzanna says, "but what really matters is that he won't have to go through what you suffered."

Say More • Not until the one-year anniversary of my third heart event, which Suzanna and I characterize as a third *attack*, when we don't know whether further damage to my heart muscle ensued despite the symptoms having been strong enough to get me in, the crew reaming out the artery (the widowmaker) and laying in two more stents; and not until we're in couples therapy with our Jungian analyst, Dr. B, our fifth session, do I register, during our fifty minutes, Suzanna's sadness, hear that "what does it take?" in her voice, meaning I remain less than fully committed to the relationship. "It's why we came to therapy," she says, anxious, edgy.

I unleash a complicated retort. The therapist, after praising my verbal agility, interrupts to say he'd like me to get to the point. He thinks I'm too much in my head. What am I driving at?

"For six years," I confess, recalling the night before, hugging Suzanna woodenly before bed, aping that bony recalcitrance my mother had, "I've been devoted more to my illness than to her. Throughout all this, I know I've let her down."

Dr. B, kindly, cool, waits while I stare out the window at a thicket of bay and eucalyptus trees on the hillside in a wooly, coastal rain before the words bass-drum out of me. I choke a bit, choosing the right ones, and he asks that I feel what I'm feeling, be honest.

"I am being honest. Aren't I?"

"What," Dr. B says, "does opening up to your letting Suzanna down feel like?"

The tree-leaf-dripping scene out the window again draws my eyes. "Oceanic," I admit.

"Say more."

"It feels like the relationship I have with my mortality is so, I don't know, personal, or private, so deep within me, between me and myself, that it's overtaken my ability to"—and I stop, aghast at the measureless Pacific across which I must sail to share this with Suzanna.

I remember a scene in Andrei Tarkovsky's film *The Sacrifice*. A man, sitting in a wood, is holding a squawking child on his lap. He says to the child, "Don't be afraid. There is no such thing as death. No. There is the fear of death, and that is an awful fear. Sometimes it even makes people do things they shouldn't. How different things would be if only we could stop fearing death!"

But it isn't just my standing on a lip of an unfathomable sea, its snotty wavelets bullying my feet.

"I have another image," I say. "I'm in a cell, jailed without cause. I'm holding the bars. Tightly. If I let the bars go they'll crumble and I'll crawl out the window. But I can't. My hands are keeping the bars in place, and I remain rigid, frozen. I want *out*, although I hold the bars in place. I'm both jailer and prisoner."

What's wrong with me? I think. Why can't I express my fear of dying like Tarkovsky's old man who tells it to a squirrelly child on his lap? Because such expression is hollow. The old man knows the child cannot understand what he's saying. Nor can he remove the child's "fear of death." The child has none. The old man is baby-sitting *his* childish fear. He's telling the child not what he wants the child to believe, but what he believes.

Suzanna disagrees that I have to abide in my prison. She says we are together so that we share what we need not face alone. "I miss your attention, your embrace, your lightness—that date we once had, dancing at a disco party, the way we were our first five years together—the foot rubs, the baths together, the side-by-side sitting on the couch. Don't you remember?"

I do. Grabbing her, mid-afternoon, for sex or pillow talk. Movie dark and head-to-head leaning. Calling her from my office just to hear her lush alto. Where had all that gone?

Just now, if I could, I would speak of my ex-wife, who once told me, though not in therapy, which we could have used and which, her words, came, maybe six months after our twin sons had been born, that she longed for the freewheeling days before, when she was "in love." Did she say "with me?" I don't remember. I doubt it. Memory, that sleeping tower guard, says her comment wasn't about me, her husband, per se, though I was the one slumped beside her on the couch, watching a made-for-TV movie with Farrah Fawcett, who connived to reclaim the buoyancy of her marriage and whose plot no doubt triggered my ex's hunger for romance. And my response? "Married people can't be 'in love,'" I said. "Not when they have children." It was, I reasoned, a cruel thing she wished for. Selfish! Our being "in love" had to evolve. It had to be transfigured into married love, the last flight off the isle of romance. Really, I countered. I was livid. *You* wanted kids. *You* badgered me until you got pregnant. After the children arrived, you wished we were "in love" more with each other and, what, less with them? And yet to my ex-wife's credit—how right she was to have wanted what she wanted, forget about blame and damage—she insisted (no, she decreed) we divorce four years later. Still, she/we had pantomimed our devotion, never "in love" again as we were that freewheeling first year. For my part, I, Mr. Responsibility, fought to hold on to our union. Why I begrudged her the freedom she sought and why I thought prolonging marriage might save us, I don't know. I couldn't leave because I was desperate, frightened of losing my kids, losing my fatherhood, and now it strikes me that this first instance of a therapy-unwrapped pattern in which I'm holding the bars of a cell in place is there so I won't face the unknown. A disease is nothing if not the unknown.

It's as though (and Dr. B is right about us verbose types: Jung was one himself) I must dive down through these movie/ex-wife allusions before I elevator to the sublevel where the therapy lies.

But then I *do* say: "I love you, Suzanna. And I hope you understand—that I couldn't rub your feet or stroke your hair as you've wanted because I've been so tightly wound in my mortality. I couldn't shake the cardiologist's words: *Did you know you were dying*? I believed *I* was supposed to know I was. Not that *we* were. My dying? I wanted to keep *that* for me."

"You can't keep that for yourself," Suzanna says. "As much as I know you want to—you can't."

"Wait—"

"Did you ever think that when the doctor asked if you knew you were dying, *I* knew you were? How do you think it felt for me to be called and told you were in the emergency room, to drive there, to see you the moment I walked in? You *were* dying. You can't change what I saw. What I felt. It *happened*. It happened to me."

I'm silent, trying to absorb her words as the hillside does the rain.

She continues. "It's just that—and this takes me back to my family, the little girl whose parents fought every night—if I tried to interfere and save my mother from my father, that only made it worse. So I shut up. They fought, and I cried. I cried and I cried and nobody ever came. So I learned to shut up. *This* is how I feel: I can't express my needs at times. I have to sit on it—and wait for someone to come."

Her eyes brim with the tears I wish I could show.

"You can't change my sharing your death," she goes on, dabbing a tissue. "It's not about what I want. It's not about what you want. It's about what's happening to *us*."

Out the window, the February rain is dripping off the hillside eucalyptus trees, the sandy ground mossy wet. Perhaps the thing I've remembered the longest about arriving in California (my first visit was at age seventeen) are those trees, their papery bark, their toasty aroma, their sun-budded insouciance. There they are, half dangling, half rising, as they've always been. The thing that links me to my initial smitten feeling about the Pacific coast, where the oceanic begins.

Where the sea starts, it also ends.

It's about what's happening to us.

A Tale of Two Haves • I'm lunching with three writer friends in San Diego. We're at the Bay Club, which overlooks a vast mooring of yachts and boats, their sails furled, their windy going stanched for now. My friends order fish, I, salad. Soon, they ask what I'm working on.

Prelude: "I've had three heart attacks," I say, and I'm met with blinkered eyes, abacks taken—*I had no idea, you seem so fit, you: unhealthy*? It's been a while since I told them, in a group email, about my first (they forgot); I haven't mentioned the shock of the second, the back-from-the-brink third.

Fugue: "I'm writing a book about my illness," for which they seem relieved, as in, illness means we avoid the pain and sorrow and go at its medical perspective. Such is the positive spin we heart patients offer to the public: focus on what's working, *not* what's not.

They tango back with questions. Three heart attacks! Family history? Prognosis? Meds? Tell us, what's the link between diet and health? Why are men vulnerable earlier and women later? For one, I say, almost all American coronary-seeking autopsies, including those of teenagers, reveal that arteriosclerosis (hardening) and stenosis (narrowing) is present. Virtually every American has a cardiovascular ailment: one in two will die of the disease.

Isn't it odd—I change direction—that we require cars to have safety restraints but we don't insist on the same in the food supply? And I don't mean USDA inspections. I mean the fat, the sugar, the additives. Why do we recall the Ford Pinto but not the Golden Corral, the Pinto of deadly food franchises? Fast food kills tens of thousands more of us than cars with fuel-tank defects or terrorists with jet planes. On like this I go, we go, to other factoids: ten percent of Medicare goes for angioplasties, etc.

I'm a flood of info. And, in response, how diffidently my companions eat. More chewing = fewer clogs. I'm spoiling their lunch.

So when one regards me with a jaundiced eye—does every meal have to be about the very meal we're eating?—I pull back.

And then a surprise drops from my mouth.

"It's the hardest piece I've ever written."

"How so?"

"The ending—not *ending* it but getting it *to* the end—is a nightmare. The book, I mean, not the life."

I confess that I used to think I would get beyond the illness, regard *beyond* silently, from a peak in Darien. But the Keatsian fantasy is not true. I've learned there is no beyond; this final phase unwraps itself only as it happens. Which, ironically, is good for the writing.

I tell my fish-eating pals, big linen napkins in their laps, about what I call the end-of-life childhood I'm in now. How its larger frame, the autobiographer's beginning-middle-end, has not coalesced. The problem is, most everything I engage as a memoirist either has been lived or is lived *in the writing*. I believe I can author this go-round *as* it happens. Call it the life-writer's conceit. Headline: "Memoirist Dies Finishing Heart Disease Story." (Little secret: for the two years it's taken to compose this book, I toyed with the subtitle, "An End to My Heart Disease." But a chronic disease ends only one way and besides, who's heart disease is it *but* mine.) I'm stuck in the confluence between writing-it and living-it. Is this the novelist's advantage, creating characters who sicken and keel over so the writer needs only to mop up?

I'm the one I'm authoring.

It's the sense you have when you eat out with friends whom you've buttonholed with so much self-ill-talk that their salad forks seem poised to stab your gesturing hand because first, they think you're well enough to write about a disease that they observe hasn't burdened you *that* much, and because second, if it had you wouldn't be writing it—you'd be stuck in bed like much of the human race, bedridden with boils and scurvy and AIDS and all the rest, so shut up and allow us to finish our halibut without having to belabor your or *our* dying.

It's the sense I have one day when Suzanna tears up; I've neglected our couch-together time (so focused am I on this book/my recovery/ the slog of dovetailing both), until, the next day, she texts, *Still lv me?*—sad, she says, she's nagged me about my attentiveness, which, she fantasizes, the day will come, and soon, when, dropping me off at the airport, she's wheel-clenching mad at my devotion to Mistress Memoir, and I board the plane, and, at twenty-seven-thousand feet up, Boom! the Boeing 747 glances the iceberg of wind, the gash is lethal, and we sink through the ocean of sky until we pancake on the Saltillo-tiled earth below.

The threat of my dying—seldom my writing about my dying—insures Suzanna's penance. I don't want to dominate my lunch friends this way. I don't want Suzanna and I to go on this way. I want it to be over, which is the it-won't-ever-be-over talking-it-over. And yet I can't help but be grateful for such a grave subject to speak on.

Yet on I go, listening to myself immerse myself in the three-ring circus of illness, unable to let the food be, unable to let the camaraderie find its footing, unable to let the little Lord Jesus, no crying he makes, be.

Its Enigmatic Nature • That the disease is something other (larger, disguised, mysterious) than the disease I've had these five years should have been apparent to me all along. But it hasn't. Its fulsomeness has *taken* time to arrive. Taken a kind of self-lacquering for me *not* to see the disease as mine but someone else's, some other self's. Taken a kind of self-orbiting for me *not* to see the disease Suzanna has seen. Taken a kind of self-enchantment for me *not* to see the illness I was convinced writing about would reveal its secrets because I'm its author-narrator-character-leading-man. Instead, the disease I have been writing about, *I* have barely felt. The writing, my doppelganger, feels it for me. (To Suzanna, I say, I worry about my heart when I *write* about my heart. That way it affects me less at other times, or so I believe.) Still, if I want to get anywhere emotionally, I must stop and feel vulnerable. I must stop what I'm doing and let myself be frightened. I must realize that the first interventional cardiologist who told me "you were dying" is as much melodramatic as it is true. I must wake up to the inadequacy of what I have felt and to the tender new sprouts I'm determined to feel. I must move out of where I want to be and travel to where I don't want to be. I can't answer why. It may be what Rumi means when he says, "The cure for the pain is in the pain."

The cure is *in* the pain. The memoirist writes now, in the gap between what was and what is, bringing what was into what is and letting what is mingle with what was. While my heart-attack symptoms are, as I type today, nearly nonexistent, I keep my heart disease *symptomatic* by writing about it.

This is why health has value, perhaps greater than it would otherwise, in the presence of disease.

This is why my not being ill remains an intimate, spooning and snuggling with my being ill, nightly bedmates with whom I'm finally getting comfortable.

Remission and Cure • Perhaps the most irritating question in philosophy concerns God the creator. To posit a creator who creates the universe is to ask, also, who created that creator. And so on and so on, a slide into oblivion Nietzsche calls Eternal Rotation. As Nick J of the "Skeptical Eye" blog argues, theists "demand an explanation for the apparent design of the universe and then postulate 'God' as their solution. . . . Atheists stop with the universe itself, as explanation is only possible within the context of existence, and therefore existence itself, the 'universe,' needs no explanation."

At some point, if you have heart disease, the gale comes, and its shipwreck is unforgettable. Once you realize that in the nature of your illness it *must* return, its coming-for-you again is just as real. But soon, via time and your psycho/medical keeping it at bay, evidence of the hour or two trauma dwindles, dries up. So what's not there is much, much bigger than what is: the absence of the infarct may be as great as the few occasions it jumps out of the bushes, scaring you senseless.

I remain locked into my own Eternal Rotation as a heart patient because another shell is always *incoming*. Even though I enjoy a year without symptoms, I still feel the need to explain to myself and others that I have a projectile roaring in, my number's up—*there*, can't you hear it? I know escape is futile, but such surety wanes when the diet is working, and the exercise is working, and the medications and the supplements are working.

So what exists seems not to exist. Its stalking me I must accept on faith—I'm certain that the longer it's away, the more likely it's due—or on the thin, vain hope that I may have beaten it.

A year after Number Three, a year of No-Oil Veganism, and a host of new tests, I'm with Dr. M in his Santa Fe office, discussing my latest numbers. He says my lipid profile is astonishing. Total cholesterol is 106 (recall it was once 261, now it's sixty percent lower); HDL, a decent 41; LDL, an extraordinary 45; triglycerides, an optimal 131 (once, 345, now sixty-two percent lower). My lipid particle count is 856, nicely below the optimal level of 1000.

"People shoot," Dr. M says, "for the eight hundreds after a heart attack, and almost never get there. With such a low particle count, [any] tendency to push cholesterol into your blood vessel wall is about zero." With my cholesterol at 106 and negligible arterial inflammation, the fairy-light dusting of cholesterol in my blood may do no harm. The test also shows I have a very low re-absorption rate of cholesterol in my bile. I'm not free of its menace but damn near.

I learn, too, that my count of 856 puts me in the bottom twenty percent of the U.S. population, some sixty million who have no heart disease. Is nonexistent the same as ended?

What's more, Dr. M says, these new tests confirm my body has "a strong tendency to pull cholesterol *out* of the blood vessel wall."

Really? What a coup!

Evidence comes first in a measure of my heart muscle fibers: those fibers, he says, "next to the damaged area of your heart, have reoriented their direction, and are working just as hard or a little less hard than they were a year ago."

I ask, Are the fibers of my dead heart muscle cells—ten to fifteen percent by my figuring—inert? What was the echocardiogram word, *akinetic*?

"Brain cells can regenerate or replace themselves," Dr. M says. "Maybe your heart cells are not as dead as we thought."

Further evidence arises from a follow-up IMT test. My intima-medial thickness, which correlates to the heart's arteries, has dropped fifteen percent. "People don't drop that much from year to year," Dr. M says.

We're not sure how much is unstable, but the reduction is significant.

What's removing the cholesterol from my artery walls? I ask.

It may be less fluid, it may be a combo of meds, it may be the artichoke extract, it may be the diet, it may be less stress. "It's all those things," Dr. M says, "moving in your favor."

Now, according to the Framingham "heart age" app, the age of my heart has fallen from sixty-eight to sixty. Heartwise, I'm sixty, younger than my present age. In the six years I've endured three heart attacks, recovered each time, been hit again, albeit less severely, and reduced the risk factors, I've *gained* eight years! A cardiovascular Benjamin Button.

Best of all, my weight has fallen from 220 to 181. Almost forty pounds gone. I'm lean again like Little League baseball.

Have I reversed the disease? How much of it is gone?

Heart disease exists when it manifests: just as the universe exists after the Big Bang manifested. (Remember, the universe existed before and during the Big Bang as well.) But when my heart disease is not there—as the numbers seem to indicate—it's at rest, a there which was lurking before, is lurking during, and will be lurking after. It is not *non*existent. Its overt evidence is gone. If the *absence* of an illness exists, then it, too, is, like a postulated God, *not there*, a useless question because no answer can be made. (What's beyond the universe? There is no beyond the universe because the universe is all we know.) And, though difficult to grok, it matters that I concentrate only on what is there, not on what is not. This, I decide, is easy for a lifelong atheist like me. And yet my health includes the disease's potential, for the disease and its penchant for hide-and-seek keeps asserting itself—the damaged heart muscle, the need for medicines, the zero cholesterol intake, the breathiness at 8500 feet, that 4 a.m. waking-up-hot.

All there.

Remission is the temporary absence of symptoms.

Which the numbers support.

Cure enters when the temporary is replaced by a permanent absence.

Which the numbers support.

In between is where I live, in the dodgy *now*: my genetic predilection and three infarcts and the accumulated cholesterol-laden muck in the arterial walls and all that cow's milk, though such muck is, I hope, decreasing (endothelial-detaching and bloodstream-disposing) via my vegan diet. So my risk is smaller than it once was, and the spacetime between remission and cure in which I finally understand how—my *body* knows how—to put this: I'm teetering toward health, which is lingering and lengthening and merging onto my track, a riderless horse I've all but caught, and when I do, all that remains for us is the finish line.

When It Happens • If you wake up with angina, it means the resting state of sleep did not calm the symptom. (Remember, angina is *not* a heart attack; it's a warning that one is coming, perhaps soon.) Rest should have calmed it. But if not, you may never know: sixty percent of nighttime heart-attack victims don't wake up. If you do awaken, take heed: a spot of nitroglycerin under the tongue should ease the pain in fifteen minutes. But if not, call 911 and tell the operator, "Heart attack," then state your address. You may gasp for air, start clapping your chest. You may drop to your knees. Don't do nothing. If the pain is bad, chew two baby aspirin, sit in a chair (don't lie down), and ask your partner or rouse a neighbor to come stay with you (partners/neighbors, please reassure the person he's going to make it—if you're frightened, he's frightened). Put the light on. If necessary, hang a towel off the screen door: Be sure the ambulance people can find you. They may save you. If you think you're blacking out, cough harshly, dramatically, to jolt the heart to keep working. If you start losing consciousness, be assured that Evolution—conspiring with Nature, that gentlest mother—often decrees you not linger.

The Sanctuary of Illness • In the simplest terms, I get to the sanctuary my illness provides once I understand my heart disease as relational, as having happened to Suzanna and me. The sanctuary is a place of protection and safety where she and I bear its acute attacks and its chronic dread. I thought the story was that it kept bedeviling *me*—and so much of this narrative speaks to that—rooted in my lineage, my weight, my diet, my destiny, a host of my's which shut down two coronary arteries, March 6, 2006. That, as they say, was only the beginning. The rest of it is waking up to the shared nature, primarily with Suzanna, of the condition. The sharing of what is ultimately not mine but ours creates the sanctuary.

The heart, too, is a sanctuary, a place where the blood, its oxygen used by muscles and organs, is re-routed into the lungs for renewed air. The heart is entombed in our chest. At that site, it's isolated, cushioned from the body's trauma when we are cut, shot, chilled, or panicked. The heart keeps pumping, keeps the body going, especially when other organs and our appendages face duress. The linings of the coronary arteries are also vulnerable, mostly to what the blood brings. But even then it takes a lot to damage those linings because they hug the heart muscle itself, bolstering their own safe haven.

The heart shares the sanctuary of the body just as Suzanna and I share my disease. The breathing our hearts support allows us sanctuary in the world. We exist because we exchange our body's carbon for the planet's oxygen in a co-replicating loop. Our breathing—alongside photosynthesis—sustains and nurtures the world.

Because of the power a heart attack has to reorient our thinking, we are unable to realize how our illness has assembled a sanctuary until after the sanctuary is up, locked in place. Erecting this haven comes as we share our condition with cardiologists, nurse practitioners, lipidologists, family, support groups, friends, loved ones: as the body *is* re-nourished, it finds a refuge in others to house its fear and its endurance.

What's also included in the sanctuary's space—a preserve, a way station, an immunity from prosecution—is room for the shadow. The dark wood where the questions, those I find most stubborn to answer, hover like harpies.

Does "heart disease" mean that my arteries at birth were robust enough to last only until I was fifty-six? At age fifty-five was my arterial *vulnerability* gene switched on and the protective sheath of the endothelia cells weakened? If the genetics are true, how did I survive all that cheese and pizza and ice cream? Why didn't I clog up at eighteen or thirty-seven? What's the most efficacious nutritional regimen that creates arteries built-to-last instead of arteries built-to-tear? If I ate stupidly, Americanly, vegetarianly, for sixty years, how might plant-based eating produce longevity, plus a healing endothelium? What is the point of a recovery if, inevitably, the disease wins? Is my recovery an end to be followed by another end, my not-recovery?

Housing a temporary fix, the sanctuary of illness also allows denial to overstay its welcome. Of the six hundred thousand people who survive an initial heart attack every year, few halt their sybaritic lifestyles, adopt a healthy diet, walk, clock in for treatment, and stabilize, beyond what the stents do, their decline. Let alone reverse *anything*. Most of this throng will (a) do nothing except take the meds and (b) suffer coronary heart disease more than they otherwise would because they have been saved from sudden death. What's coming? The list is not pretty. A second or third heart attack, bypass surgery and its complications, pulmonary embolisms, the dying of more heart-muscle cells, which often leads to cardiomyopathy and congestive heart failure.

Despite its wearing away, the heart is *for* us even when we're not for it. In the denial-ridden, overweight patient, a sluggish, failing heart pumps oxygen-rich blood to the body's cells as it always has. If the body receives less blood to its cells and organs and tissues, the heart works harder to tunnel the necessary pathways (the medical term is vascularize) to deliver blood. Such, Sherwin Nuland writes in *How We Die*, is the heart's cycle of failure—"a kind of vicious circle of [the heart's] trying to disguise its own inadequacies by straining to compensate for them."

Perfect, *that cross.*

Such is the bighearted ambiguity of *sanctuary.*

After I'd been stented three times for my first heart attack, my second and third infarcts were less severe: my blood was sliding through the tiny chromium culverts that rimmed the site of my first plaque rupture. Stent technology lessens the severity of later attacks whose unimpeded flow tricks you into thinking you're fixed. Each stent re-bloods you, and the bloodedness makes you less aware, forgetful—mercifully forgetful—of your condition.

Another (perfect) cross, the illusion-filled music of health.

The most important thing I've had to learn came, as my father would have put it, *the hard way*. That the awareness the blood keeps diminishing and expanding in me is how it's supposed to be.

The day after the body tries and fails to end the body's reign—easily, the deadliest attack you've faced—you believe you are invincible.

The week after when you feel your life has been saved and given its (temporary) sanctuary—and nothing will ever equal that feeling—is when you begin to challenge its domain.

In your sanctuary, you enlist a partner who helps you sort it out, mirror its conundrums, accept its enigmas, for you can't do all that yourself, I don't care how wily and willful you are.

Then you notice an escape valve—room just outside the sanctuary (perhaps at the edge of the universe) where you might also abide, happily unaware of it all.

Both places are borderless and secure. Both are home.

And swinging to-and-fro between in-it and out-of-it, my fellow heart patient, is as simple a case as I can make.

In Santa Fe • At the end of May, 2012, Suzanna and I spend a day devoted to being together. We hug and remark about how close we feel. She says, kissing me goodnight, that no doubt many muzzy days lie ahead, this one's a Red Giant and glows with grandiosity. It starts with our Sunday ritual, the *New York Times*, my devouring eight or so of the essays in the "Sunday Review," her an equal amount in the "Book Review" or "Style" or "Art & Leisure." Post-coffee, breakfast granola with blueberries and strawberries, we plant-eaters are verging on slender. Soon we're shopping at the outlet stores where she buys a stack of shirts/shoes/pants and I a jacket, a shirt, two pairs of socks. The more mundane the pleasanter it tacks—such a seaworthy lift, clear Southwest sky, seventy degrees, billowing sails, no drought-tendered fires or smoky gray-outs yet. Back in town, at Whole Foods, we load $300 worth of greens, fruit, deli stuff, cereals, bottles of supplements, Francis Ford Coppola wine. We remember our bags. Home, unload clothes and groceries. Naps. Then to crown the day, one of us raises the fine idea around five-thirty—sex.

Seven years ago, before sex—two from San Diego, staying in a Hollywood hotel—he got out of the shower, swaddled himself in a towel, and brushed his teeth before the movie-close-up mirror. Pre-heart attack, he never looked at his waist—a waste of time since he knew he was tubbing up just like his dad and his brother. He avoided gyms, scales, physicals, anything where he had to weigh in. Don't look. This time he did. And there it was. A distended hump, a midriff donut, whose plumpness supported his breasts, flabby cones lying like wedges atop his bulge. A regular Ron Jeremy. *Shit*, that was ugly. Why would she want him, in bed or otherwise? The body admired is the body loved. He couldn't stand before her, self-consciously protuberant. He robed, rushed to the bed, turned away from her, dropped the toga, and slid under the covers. His desire flown, his penis limp, he tried, he tried—thrice he tried—then sulked in his corner. She shook him, saying, "It doesn't matter, honey. We'll go another time."

Today, my fat fled, my ailment caved, my lust, alas, still needs a boost. I chew the blue pill, wait an hour, and it's here again, the wild-fire, the finger in the outlet, skin galvanic at first, then the pulsing neurotic tremors in my lower depths, my gonads, my crotch—not exactly a Napoleonic surge in my cock but rather a field-tent set-to between the cannoneer and me, readying for the campaign, bombs at first light. Snuffling goatishly, I feel a pair of Matterhorns pro-trude out my forehead.

First, though, we shower, soap genitals, brush teeth; at my request, she dons underwear, and we fling the covers back, snuggle, rub, kiss, hump, stroke, moan-a-lot, talk dirty (at least I do). We ogle each other briefly. I don't mind being seen now, and Suzanna enjoys being dominated, though she asks/expects it so willingly there's really no prey to cage. She's quite self-directed with her six-setting, double "D," Jack Rabbit vibrator, a pink plastic rubber-molded authentification of a penis (alas, not mine). A device with which she, but not before I caress and squeeze and suck on her tits for ten minutes, nuzzles that shaking-embracive fork onto her clit and shouts her way up the mountain, getting off in body-flapping waves of agonal pleasure like Mario and Tosca's Act 1 duet. (The neighbors, we laugh, have ceased watering the garden and are listening in.) She says it's me. I say it's the vibrator. She needs no pill. I do. Ms. Eveready. Mr. Catch-up. Thanks to Pfizer, Viagra relaxes the blood vessels in my penis so it can fill with blood. But the blood's got to get down there. Thus, the joy of post-infarct arterial remodeling—rushing the blood with unimpeded passion to its target and activating, once again, our shared wantonness, the most primal of the many things that drew Suzanna and me together all those years ago.

I'm grateful for this lingering lasciviousness; I don't care that it comes with a miracle chemical surge. (As my partner often says, "I like having sex—with you.") It's a sweet state we share, in addition to our genital charge. I have wanted to feel this again: that I am/we are *almost* as I was/we were before. I know Suzanna will not air her full-fathom fear that my infarct-ridden core will one day just quit. I know my disease's authoritarian rule will never end for her—that my dying, so far, trumps hers. I know her son's condition (he's maintaining; the monthly statin-drug infusion, working) weighs heavy as well; she may outlast her two dearest males. I also recognize some exaggeration (a self-regard; a partnership-regard) in these passages I write and revise. But, at least, I've unloosed the ambiguity every heart-heavy incident, remembered exactly as it happened or recast by the survivor's emotion, insists I bear.

Life is but a dream, goes the nursery rhyme.

But what is life dreaming of?

Of being alive.

As we are, just now.

Suzanna's head rests on my chest and her hand strokes my stomach. My hand crawls under the small of her back, and our postcoital breathing is like water lapping at a boat's hull, oceanworthy passengers adrift on a shipless sea. In the tempestuous quiet, we float to that familiar isle where our hearts, when we awaken, are beating still.

ACKNOWLEDGMENTS

I'm grateful to Joe Mackall and Dan Lehman of *River Teeth* who published "Disenthralled: An End to My Heart Disease," a long hybrid essay that marked this book's first gestation. I thank Dinty Moore, who took a 750-word description of my first heart attack, called "One Way It Happens," for *Brevity*, January 2013. I'm gratified that Kristen Radtke showed my video essay, "I'm Sorry / What For?" a love song to my partner, Suzanna, at the 2013 AWP conference in Boston. I appreciate the editors at *The Yale Journal for Humanities in Medicine,* who published "Stress Echo" in June 2013. And I treasure my colleagues and our students in the Ashland University MFA program in creative nonfiction for their interest in my PowerPoint-accompanied reading about my illness at the college in 2011.

Barrels of thanks to readers of the work-in-progress as well as to those who consoled me during my recent, rough days: Elizabeth Raby, Richard Buch, Steve Harvey, Richard Keith, John Abel, Tom Adler, Shel Neymark, Liz Riedel, Michael and Carole Steinberg, Peggy Frailey, Betsy Hurley, Carolyn Angell, Joan Mangan, Tom and Kay Sanger, Jane Lipman, Bill Rosen, Clare Adrian, Jay Hasheider, my men's group—Marc Lampe, John Christiansen, Dale Barbour, Mark Linsky, and the late Bob O'Neil—and my sons, Jeremy and Blake Larson. I'm indebted to the cardiology staffs at Scripps Green Hospital in La Jolla, California, and at Lancaster General Hospital in Lancaster, Pennsylvania, for saving me so effortlessly. Kudos to my attentive, down-to-earth lipidologist, Jim Mickle, in Santa Fe, New Mexico; to Mike Cobble, M.D., for writing a fine appreciation of my book; to my neighbor Erik Olson for a bunch of fine photographs;

to my buddy, the filmmaker John Eddy, for a video interview and film of Suzanna and me; and to the maintenance crew of the Faith and John Meem Library at St. John's College in Santa Fe, where, with its summertime air-conditioning, its exceptional stock of classic books, and its spotty Internet connection, the bulk of this memoir was written.

As for authorial influences. Three memoirists and their books—*Half a Life*, Darrin Straus; *The Two Kinds of Decay*, Sarah Manguso; *Resisting Elegy*, Joel Peckham—taught me to intensify the gravest and most intimate moments of my illness and to quicken all else, whether narrative or reflective. I hope such focus and acceleration create the momentum that moves the story and compels the reading.

Hudson Whitman / Excelsior College Press is fortunate to have the gracious Sue Petrie as its director and the talented William Patrick as its editor, both of whose intelligent suggestions improved the book. They have made editing, publishing, and marketing this memoir a joy.

The following resources have been crucial for my learning about my condition: *Prevent and Reverse Heart Disease* by Dr. Caldwell Esselstyn (whose phone calls I appreciate as well as his advice to eat six fistfuls of greens every day); *The China Syndrome* by C. Colin Campbell; *The Starch Solution* by Dr. John McDougall; the heart-healthy films, *Forks Over Knives*, *Fat, Sick and Nearly Dead*, and *Escape Fire*; and the vegan recipes in *The Cancer Survivor's Guide: Foods That Help You Fight Back* by Drs. Neal Barnard and Jennifer K. Reilly. Barnard's Physicians Committee for Responsible Medicine (www.pcrm.org) is a great organization for those who want to use food to avoid the causes and combat the consequences of many diseases.

I wish again to acknowledge Suzanna, who verified the conversations between us that populate this memoir. She has been an insightful reader and editor of the experiences I render, especially the dramatic highs and lows we have shared. Every writer should be as lucky as I have to spend half his life with a person who loves me for who I am and supports me in what I do: neither this book nor my freewheeling writing life would be possible without her. There is always a musical equivalent for our deepest feelings, those we try to express with words. One set of my feelings for Suzanna is captured in the song "River Road" by Jimmy LaFave.

Finally, let me advise the eighteen million Americans with coronary artery disease with a few ideas that extend to partners, children, and relatives who wish to support them. To prolong life and suffer heart disease less, you will benefit if you 1) stop consuming meat and dairy; 2) eat lots of green leafy vegetables; and 3) walk every day. These three changes will help you lose belly fat. The correlation is real: the fat around your waist is the fat that has clogged your arteries. Everyone who has any heart malady should consult a cardiologist and/or a lipidologist for a health plan, including a lipid profile. With the three things I suggest, your LDL cholesterol drops, your coronary arteries become less inflamed and less threatened by vulnerable plaques, and you feel younger. During recovery, a doctor's part is smaller than you think. Most changes are your responsibility. Only you can unleash the power of nutrition. Only you can advocate for your health.

On my website, www.thomaslarson.com, I maintain updates about my health—my eating and exercise regimens, my cholesterol numbers, and my supplements. My greatest discovery about a plant-based diet is that if being overweight or obese is a problem—and it is for many Americans; it certainly was for me—a plant-based diet solves it. Most everyone who eats fruits, vegetables, legumes, and whole-wheat starches do not put on the pounds. Best of all, you can eat as much as you like, and you will never have to diet again.

ABOUT THE AUTHOR

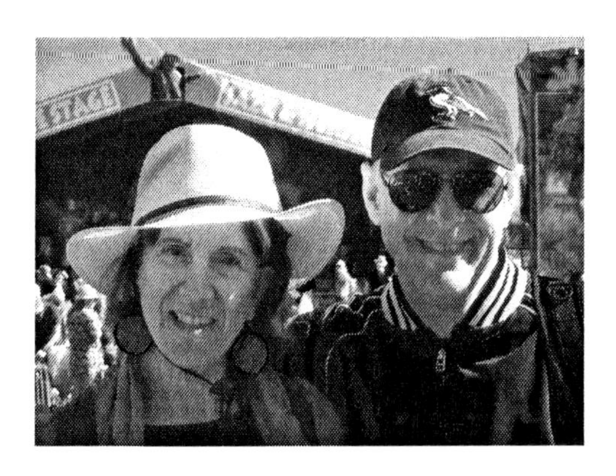

Suzanna Neal and the author,
May 1, 2013, New Orleans Jazz & Heritage Festival

Journalist, critic, and memoirist, Thomas Larson has been a staff writer for the *San Diego Reader* for fifteen years. His books include *The Memoir and the Memoirist* (Swallow Press) and *The Saddest Music Ever Written: The Story of Samuel Barber's* "Adagio for Strings" (Pegasus Books). His work has appeared in dozens of publications, among them *Oxford American*, *Antioch Review*, *New Letters*, *Missouri Review*, *TriQuarterly*, *River Teeth*, and the *Los Angeles Review of Books*. He teaches in the low-residency MFA program in creative nonfiction at Ashland University, Ashland, Ohio.

Larson is available for speaking engagements, book clubs, and writing workshops—especially to medical communities—based on this book. He offers a PowerPoint presentation on heart disease and a writing workshop, "Writing About Illness," which can be adapted for nurses, doctors, patients, and medical administrators as well as participants in narrative and integrative medicine programs. Please see his website, www.thomaslarson.com, for more information.

ABOUT HUDSON WHITMAN

Hudson Whitman is a new, small press affiliated with Excelsior College, which has administrative offices in Albany, New York.

Our tagline is "Books That Make a Difference," and we aim to publish high-quality nonfiction books and multimedia projects in areas that complement Excelsior's academic strengths: education, nursing, health care, military interests, business and technology, with one "open" category, American culture and society.

If you would like to submit a manuscript or proposal, please review the guidelines on our website, hudsonwhitman.com. Feel free to send a note with any questions. We endeavor to respond as soon as possible.

OTHER TITLES BY HUDSON WHITMAN

The Call of Nursing: Stories from the Front Lines of Health Care
William B. Patrick (print and e-book)

Shot: Staying Alive with Diabetes
Amy Ryan (print and e-book)

The Language of Men: A Memoir
Anthony D'Aries (print and e-book)
2012 ForeWord Book of the Year Gold - Autobiography

Courageous Learning:
Finding a New Path through Higher Education
John Ebersole and William Patrick (print and e-book)

Saving Troy:
A Year with Firefighters and Paramedics in a Battered City
William Patrick (e-book only)